ENDORSE

"Shannon Green's thorough research a̱ answer for Guillain-Barre is truly inspiring in terms of understanding its complexity ͙ͅcome a better teacher. She also truly cares abouͳ ͙ͅ ͙ͅers through her numerous resources and connections. Her journey and experience will give you all the tools needed to start your pain management journey."

—**Pree Poonati,** yoga/personal trainer

"This book is full of hacks to help heal your body and mind. As a massage therapist, I have gained new knowledge for the treatment of chronic pain. Also, that the road to healing is a long one but with the help of the "Chronic Pain Hacker" there are many ways to find what will work for the individual. And not to give up when the pain is too much."

—**Amber C.,** LMT

"I am honored to have worked with Shannon over the past year and her service to the chronic pain community with sharing wise choices hard won. I am both moved by her story of recovery and a witness to her healing journey. Having suffered with auto-immune dysfunction myself, her wonderful attitude and message is the voice of a needed navigator. Thank you Shannon!"

—**Michael Parrish,** LMT

"We know Shannon through our monthly Chronic Pain Support Group meetings. We share news, views, articles, information, what works for us and what doesn't, as well as coffee and donuts! I greatly admire Shannon and wish I could learn to gain the same wisdom and insight to control my pain as she has done."

—**Janet and Gary Tracy,** ACPA support group members

"Shannon suffers from chronic pain syndrome but with the help of physical therapy, at Apex Manual Therapy, she was able to gain more control over her pain. Shannon learned to recognize and correct faulty movement patterns that were contributing to her pain. After completing physical therapy, Shannon was able to take a more active role in her family's life."

—**Alicia Shugart, PT, DPT, FAAOMP**
Fellow of the American Academy of Orthopedic Manual Physical Therapists

Fearless (6x9) Self-Publishing Template © 2017 Renee Fisher
https://www.reneefisher.com

Cover Design: by Nelly Murariu at PixBeeDesign.com

ISBN-13: 978-0-578-67322-6
ISBN-10: 0-578-67322-3

Chronic Pain

Hacker

Because Healing is Hard

SHANNON GREEN

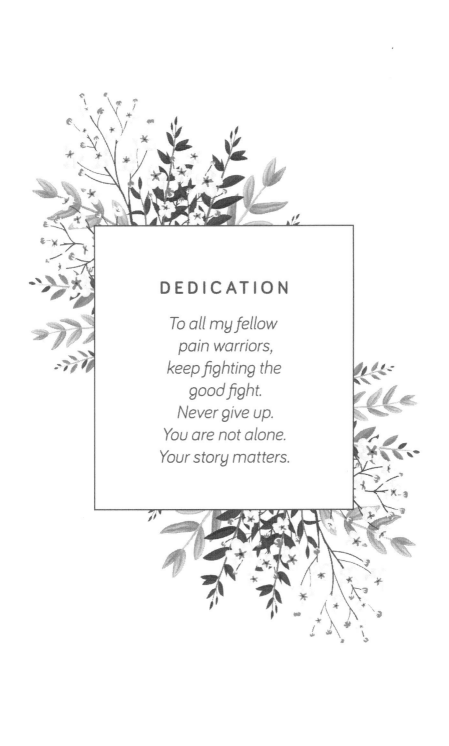

DEDICATION

*To all my fellow
pain warriors,
keep fighting the
good fight.
Never give up.
You are not alone.
Your story matters.*

TABLE OF CONTENTS

INTRODUCTION

*T*his book offers some practical advice on the latest therapeutic and diagnostic advances as well as lifestyle modifications to improve the lives of those diagnosed with long-term chronic pain. Furthermore, I want to highlight the development of tools and skills that are essential life lines that can change the trajectory of life. Family and friends play a large role as a support system so it's important to include them in this process.

I want to introduce the connection between emotional trauma and physical pain. The link between unresolved trauma and physical pain is considerable. In my case, trauma was running in the background like an application open on the desktop but not properly closed. Years of trauma accumulation can lead to the concept of the "pain body".

My journey dealing with chronic pain goes back over thirty-five years. Subsequently, my expertise focuses on the areas of neuropathy, back pain, fibromyalgia, depression, anxiety, Guillain-Barre Syndrome (GBS) pronounced gee-YAN-bah-RAY, epilepsy, and psychogenic nonepileptic seizures (PNES).

Prior to writing this book, I was a technical writer of accounting software and processes at such large corporations as Verizon and IBM. Therefore, I have divided up the chapters based on quick search topics and resources using this format style. Interesting stories are weaved in to compliment the technical portion and provide compelling action.

I received several awards for my work. I worked in the accounting industry for 15 years. I despised the tedious part of accounting but was fascinated with how my research could lead to the automation of manual processes. These awards accompanied by my masters of business administration (MBA) qualified me for a rare opportunity.

This opportunity was in the law enforcement industry. Shortly after 9/11, I applied to the Federal Bureau of Investigation (FBI) to be a special agent. Never in a million years did I expect to get selected out of 35 thousand applicants for an interview. I passed the written test, lie detector test, background check, and the fitness test. This was over a span of two years. Ultimately, I was not selected due to health issues like back pain, exercise induced asthma, and history of depression.

Most of my work was based on process improvement. Most of these years were in a project management role rather than a number cruncher. I still use this "research" approach to tackle things in my personal life. This spark was the catalyst for this book.

My hope is that this book equips you with enough information to make very important decisions about your health and overall wellness. If you're looking for a magic pill or a quick fix solution then this is not the book for you.

The journey to wellness is a slow process of trial and error. You have to be willing to do the work. "Nothing great comes easy, and nothing easy can ever equate to greatness." Edmond Mbiaka

Despite this, I share my experience navigating medical and holistic practices so that some of you might not have to reinvent the wheel. I have put in thousands of dollars and man hours researching as many treatments, medications, and supplements as possible. I hope it will help improve the quality of my life and yours.

In recent years the growth of the holistic marketplace provides some nontraditional approaches for dealing with pain and nutrition. Whole Foods opened the door for the supplement market to take off. They are the hipster version of General Nutrition Centers (GNC) that were located in suburban indoor shopping malls across America in the 1980's. Now, they are mostly located in outdoor shopping centers with other anchor stores like Target.

An integrated (functional) approach can be more effective because it merges the best options from both worlds. It's my opinion that a combined approach gives us more options for healing. Therefore, when the limitations of western medicine present no cure, or a bleak long-term diagnosis, holistic living approaches can provide some much needed relief and hope.

It's a coordinated effort that requires planning and implementation. In a perfect world, a primary care doctor is on board with an integrated approach and communicates with other specialists about a patient's overall health. For example, my psychiatrist sends a copy of our session notes to my primary doctor so that everyone is on the same page.

Furthermore, I am not a doctor or nurse so the opinions expressed in this book are based on my own personal experience. Consult your doctor before trying a new supplement or service. I have had the opportunity to visit numerous doctors all over the U.S. I had some real conversations with them about chronic pain management. This forged the relationship with several foundations and advocacy groups.

My goal is to fight for patient advocacy for those affected by chronic pain. I want to volunteer with organizations like, U.S. Preventive Services Task Force, American Chronic Pain Association (ACPA), and GBS-CIDP Foundation. I want to leave this world a better place. I believe I can encourage individuals to lead their best life. The goal is to reduce suffering and increase balance in all areas of life.

Together we can propose and chase important legislation that will improve the lives of many Americans. Example topics include:

management of opioid crisis, marijuana legislation, insurance plans that are not tied to employment, and adding coverage of massage and acupuncture to all health care insurance plans.

Also, what if we can teach the next generation how to handle adversity, stress, illness and break the generational cycle of pain? Millennials will especially need this because they have grown up with social media, smartphones, video games, and the internet.

Scientists are currently studying the long term effects of this trend. Furthermore, many Americans are "numbing out" on these devices for hours every day. What does this do to our mental and physical health?

We have the opportunity to pass on healthy coping mechanisms. For example, my grandmother, grandfather, father, and myself all have mental issues of some sort that were passed down to generation after generation.

More importantly, healthcare is expensive and there are so many treatment options, services, meds, and supplements, it's overwhelming. Each year, healthcare premiums are on the rise. According to Electronic Health Reporter, "Health care spending is expected to reach $8.7 trillion by 2020."[1]

Alternative treatments can be expensive. On average, they range from $60-100 U.S. dollars per hour for services like acupuncture, chiropractic, and massage. Also, mental health services like "talk therapy" are usually over $100 per hour. It can be very overwhelming with the various choices of therapy, not to mention selecting a competent provider. Finding a therapist that is accepting new patients is difficult.

Lastly, chronic pain of a physical and mental nature are discussed. I hope to reduce the stigma of mental illness. We as a society need to shed some light on those topics that are difficult to talk about.

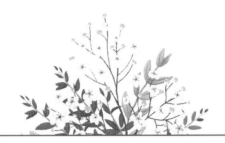

Grace, Gratitude, and Guillain-Barre (GBS)

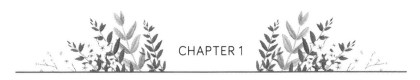

CHAPTER 1

DOCTORS

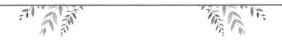

*T*here is a shortage of primary care doctors in the U.S., making it difficult to find same-day appointments. Therefore, the trend has been an increase in emergency room (ER) and or urgent care visits in the U.S. This has caused overcrowding in ERs across the U.S., causing some patients to wait over ten hours to see a doctor.

How can doctors equip their patients with the knowledge to decipher when something is a real emergency? What if doctors and patients come up with an emergency plan so that precious time isn't wasted? For example, for chronic conditions, doctors can distinguish between what is a flare and what is an emergency.

Pain flares are notoriously seen as an emergency by the patient. I have been there. The feeling like you might die unless you get immediate assistance. I have asked my doctor many times whether something is a real emergency. He/she can offer suggestions of things you might try first before seeking emergency care.

Another clog in the system is the quality of the relationship between a provider and the patient. Sometimes, many of us feel we are "stuck" with a doctor because it's hard to find another doctor quickly. I fell victim to this mentality.

Now, that I am a seasoned veteran of doctor visits, I can't afford the time and money to keep paying a doctor that I feel is not helping me. I have felt like just a number on many occasions while waiting in a provider's waiting room.

I have fired many doctors and searched for a second, third, or fourth opinion. I actually told a neurologist, "Humans can put a man on the moon but you are telling me my only hope is an expensive pill with terrible side effects every day for the rest of my life. What else do you recommend?" When he replied, "Nothing." I stormed out of his office stating that I would never be back.

I no longer go to a pain management clinic because I felt they weren't really helping me. They had me on numerous medications where I could barely hold up my head. The brain fog was so intense on these medications that I could barely function.

The other trend is that doctors are treating just the tip of the iceberg because taking the time to thoroughly research the root problem of an illness requires too much time and money. This isn't supported in our current U.S. healthcare environment.

Many doctors are pressured by insurance companies to see as many patients as possible. Fifteen minutes is the average length of a doctor visit in the U.S. The doctors that spend the extra time with their patients are rewarded with overflowing waiting rooms. They get backed up and the wait time increases and their day just got longer.

This causes a band-aid approach to diagnosis and the over prescribing of medications. Many treatments or medications are masking the real problem instead of treating the root cause. In many cases, it's hard to tell if the symptoms are real or stem from the side effects of medications.

It's a scary trial and error process. Many medications take a minimum of 90 days before you receive the full effect. In some cases a person may not have 90 days to wait.

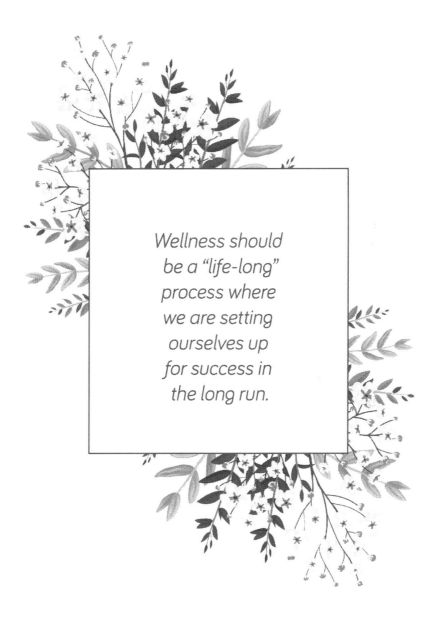

Wellness should be a "life-long" process where we are setting ourselves up for success in the long run.

My primary care doctor left a big corporate company to start his own practice. This way he is able to provide quality care on his terms. Also, he offers more affordable options for his patients. He is also able to spend more time with each patient. He spends on average an hour with me on each visit. He also offers affordable prices that are posted, which is especially important for making the decision to use insurance or not for a certain type of treatment or procedure. He even offers plans for the uninsured patient.

Furthermore, I think there should be a doctor/patient interview process before a patient officially selects a doctor to be their primary care doctor. Questions like, "Do you prefer to offer holistic solutions at first try or is a pill prescribed at the first mention of a symptom?" "How do you feel about a patient asking for a new med by name instead of waiting for the doctor to explain the options?" "Are you a medical doctor (M.D.) or Doctor of Osteopathic Medicine (D.O.)? As a D.O., can you provide spinal manipulations?" "Are your rates for services posted online or somewhere visible in the office?"

In my experience, D.O.'s usually practice integrative medicine meaning they usually suggest alternative options like diet and exercise before prescribing medication. However, this isn't always the case, that is why I think it's important to ask these questions up front regardless of the doctor's title of D.O. or M.D.

Fortunately, another trend is on the rise. It's "telemedicine." Telemedicine provides a video visit with your doctor over a secure application. I have had it for two years, and it's amazing! For patients who can't drive, or who have difficulty driving like myself, this is revolutionary. During the Coronavirus outbreak of 2020, many doctors offered video conference appointments for the first time.

Telemedicine can provide access to your doctor 24/7. In 2019, I paid $150/year for telemedicine care from my primary doctor.

It's worth every penny and then some. The peace of mind that my doctor is just a text, video, or phone call away is amazing. This is especially important when a patient has a complicated medical history that would be difficult to explain to a new doctor.

To elaborate further, I think doctors should give patients an actual Rx on their prescription pad for exercise and or healthy meal plan suggestions. This Rx should be placed in a visible place like in the kitchen or the bathroom mirror to remind us to commit to lifestyle modifications as a real lifestyle change, not just the next fad diet or goat yoga.

Wellness should be a" life-long" process where we are setting ourselves up for success in the long run. I know this is easier said than done. I have failed at the healthy eating plans so many times that I have lost track. I have failed at getting thirty minutes of daily exercise consistently and used the excuse that my pain was too bad.

Moreover, in the long run, our bodies will hurt more if we don't get up and move. A sedentary lifestyle only adds to musculoskeletal issues. It can set up a life long pain relationship with our bodies that takes its toll on the back, neck, and joints.

This book outlines many treatments, services, supplements, meds, etc. with a brief description of the advantages and disadvantages. My hope is that this information will help guide your decision making in choosing the most cost-effective and beneficial solution for you.

I want to challenge people to seek out a customized treatment plan that is tailor made for your mind, body, and soul. I think it's important for a doctor to know your routine in areas like exercise, yoga, deep breathing, counseling, meditation, and other lifestyle enhancements.

Also, make sure your doctor has a list of supplements, vitamins, and other OTC medications you take in order to avoid a possible drug interaction. It's also helpful to get your medications filled at the same pharmacy so the pharmacist can check for drug interactions.

If possible, have all medications prescribed by one doctor. I have had several bad drug interactions that caused me to end up in the hospital. I had to develop this policy. This creates a two-tier check and balance system. This system can not only identify possible medication allergies but it can also flag those meds that don't work well together.

A valuable life hack I have discovered is documentation. Ensure all visits with various doctors and practitioners are well documented on both the patient's part and that of the doctor's medical records. Keep a journal of your doctor visits with dates, medication changes, and items discussed. I keep a binder and include blood work labs, x rays, etc.

This is helpful when, five years down the road, a doctor asks you if you have tried "XYZ" medication. This way reliance on faulty memory to remember some long and weird sounding medication is limited. Also, use Google to look up the generic and brand name of a medication. Different parts of the world use different names for the same medication. I promise you that this will save you time, expense, and worry.

When looking for a doctor, check online reviews before your appointment. "Vitals" is the largest online database of patient reviews for doctors and facilities. Also, check out doctor reviews at the following sites below:

www.vitals.com

www.healthgrades.com

www.topdoctors.com

www.ratemds.com

Doctors find chronic pain difficult to treat for a number of reasons.

Similarly, Stacey Colino talks about chronic pain in her article, *"Tuning Out Pain"* in *Brain and Mind* magazine ,"She explains how chronic pain doesn't go away but treating it wisely and learning to live with it can alter its intensity. Researchers are beginning to recognize that there is not a single mechanism for chronic pain; it's a cascade of events."[2]

Consequently, it's important to note that the healthcare industry has a big incentive to *"keep"* people sick. It's a billion dollar industry and money is to be made by selling medications, supplements, vitamins, services, and doctor appointments. If I had a dollar for every time I saw a pharmaceutical sales rep go ahead of me in line at the doctor's office, I would be a rich lady.

Let's not forget the commercials that say, "Ask your doctor if XYZ medicine is right for you." Drug companies are marketing directly to patients. They provide incentives for doctors to prescribe expensive medications with terrible side effects, but show a happy person walking in the park with their dog in the advertisement.

We, as humans, expect to have a *"one magic pill"* solution to our problem. Many times, doctors are throwing medications at symptoms instead of trying to find the real, root cause of the problem. To their credit, a fifteen minute doctor visit is not enough time to properly diagnose a complicated medical condition, especially one that has persisted for decades.

We don't want to do "the work" required to actually fix the root problem. It's so much easier and quicker to just take a pill. This strategy works well in the short term but in the long term, it can have dire consequences.

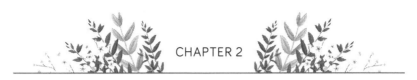

CHAPTER 2

CHRONIC PAIN

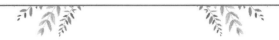

*T*here are many stressors that contribute to chronic pain. For example, there were thirty-five years of events and trauma that led up to my current "pain body." Examples of these events are: car wrecks, poor posture, unresolved trauma, sexual assault, bi-polar parent, alcoholic parent, death of parents and in-laws, bad falls, failed surgeries, and years of eleven hour days slumped over a computer in corporate America.

Stacey Colino continues to explain how pain works, "As the central nervous system becomes increasingly sensitized to pain, there's a failure of pain-inhibiting mechanisms (cells in the brain and spinal cord), that promote inflammation, and stress hormones also play a role. Changes in wiring occur in the brain, and the mechanisms become ingrained in the nervous system.

The phenomenon of chronic pain is often compared to a faulty alarm system. Without good reason, the siren continuously goes off, and it may take less and less to trip the wiring, causing the pain to flare, especially as we age. In addition, how people respond to pain affects how they experience it." [2]

Despite this, I believe in my soul that everything happens for a reason, and that God is using my voice to help others in pain. This is not a religious book, but I firmly believe in the Bible verse,

Romans 8:28 King James Version, "And we know that all things work together for good to those who love God, to those who are the called according to His purpose."[3]

In other words, God has your back. He has a purpose for your life. His will is probably not going to reveal itself like a large, neon sign, but He does have His methods of revealment. As a child, I used to pray for this big, neon sign that would be so obvious I was sure not to miss it. Oftentimes, He does reveal himself to us, but we aren't in the right "headspace" to comprehend, or we are so distracted by life that we miss the subtle signs.

More importantly, a bleak, long-term diagnosis is devastating and overwhelming for the patient and their family. Caring for a loved one with chronic pain changes the family dynamic forever. I started asking myself, "Is this all there is...was I made for more?...I expected more out of life, right, I deserve more? I feel like a burden to my family...do they resent me?"

The intensity of chronic pain can be dialed down by incorporating many holistic approaches and services. For example, meditation is one of the easiest to incorporate. My daily recommendation for meditation is 20-30 minutes. Meditation alters the brain's function in a positive way, decreasing pain, improving focus and memory, mood improvement, and assists with the effects of aging. Start out slow with just five minutes of meditation/day even if that means just sitting in a dark and quiet room with no distractions and your eyes closed.

There are many mindfulness meditation apps like "Calm" at www.calm.com and "Headspace" at www.headspace.com that can send reminders and even offer guided meditation or relaxing sounds. Meditation assists the brain with overactivity, which can slow down the pain messages.

The amount of products, supplements, specialist recommendations, medications, and services available blow my mind. They can be expensive, confusing, time-consuming, and full of unwanted side effects. Every expert has an opinion on what you should or should not do after only meeting you for thirty minutes.

The last thing a chronically ill person wants to hear is that they need to move more. Also, many folks will ask questions like, "Have you tried yoga? Have you tried an all plant based diet or keto?" These questions are overwhelming.

Healthy folks don't realize the amount of energy it takes just to perform basic tasks like walking, grooming, or going to the bathroom. I feel like screaming at that nosy and not-so-helpful person, "I'm fighting for every step I take to remain upright and walk across a room or it takes a lot of effort to make this magic happen."

Every step is a battle between fatigue, nerve and muscle damage, pain, and fear. "No, I can't go walking with you for leisure because I must store up my energy for the steps that are mandatory." I try not to voice these snarky thoughts out loud. I have to think to myself, "inside or outside voice."

There are those well-meaning souls who comment about my ability to perform a task or ask why I parked in a handicap parking spot when I don't *"look sick"*. The amount of time required to schedule, drive, wait in the waiting room, and see a doctor is very time consuming, much more than folks realize.

My therapist advises me not to waste my time explaining my disability and or condition. She says, "They aren't going to get it so don't waste your breath." Many of us have invisible illnesses like fibromyalgia, for example. We don't look sick but that doesn't mean we aren't.

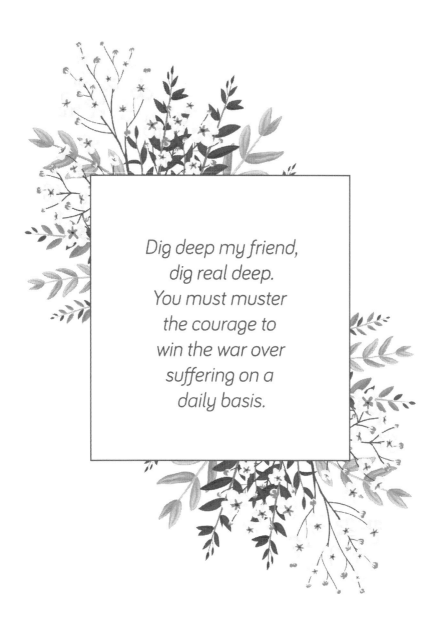

*Dig deep my friend,
dig real deep.
You must muster
the courage to
win the war over
suffering on a
daily basis.*

For example, fibromyalgia is not always taken seriously as a valid diagnosis because it doesn't have a definitive diagnostic test. I have been living with fibromyalgia since 2009 and I can confirm that it's real and absolutely devastating.

Furthermore, my condition is none of their business, and what others think of me is none of my business. This truth is a game changer. This might be the secret to a happy life. I learned to stop caring what others think. This is so hard. I fail sometimes, but I try to practice this concept daily and not focus on the "what ifs". Life is too short to worry.

Gym trainers, physical therapists, holistic providers, etc. are well meaning but when they comment on my obesity, I have a panic attack. I feel like saying, "Gee, I didn't realize I'm fat but thanks for letting me know." These statements made me feel even more depressed because I felt like a failure for being overweight my whole life. Shame is a powerful thing and can be quite destructive.

They begin to profess how much better my life would be if I just ate healthy or tried an all plant diet. Again, I want to say, "If it was that easy for me, I would have already figured it out." It's frustrating because the reason I eat unhealthy and or binge eat is because of my fear, depression, and anxiety, not because I don't know how to eat healthy.

The thought of just putting a meal plan together gives me panic, not to mention the grocery shopping and actual preparation of the meal. However, now that my groceries are delivered, it gives me more time to focus on the meal prep. Grocery delivery is life changing!

Expectations play a big role in chronic pain management. Unrealistic expectations can lead to anxiety, grief, and depression when the "miracle cure" doesn't work or come to fruition. Suffering is increased, when expectations are not met. A wise therapist gave me this formula for "radical acceptance". I placed the notecard in a strategic viewing place like my mirror, car, or white board.

> **PAIN WITH NON-ACCEPTANCE = SUFFERING**
>
> **PAIN WITH ACCEPTANCE = JOY**

Radical acceptance is not: approval, compassion, love, passivity, or against change. I found it helpful to focus on a statement of acceptance such as "It is what it is." Suffering occurs when unmet expectations cause us to grieve when things don't work out the way we planned or dreamed they would. "Expectations are the thief of joy." Theodore Roosevelt

In addition, let go of the "shoulds" and let things be as they are. A sense of entitlement clouds the picture, and as humans, we inherently believe we deserve to be completely healthy and happy. This disconnection between reality and our expectations is the root of suffering. The goal is to reduce suffering. The reduction of suffering is a more meaningful goal than just stating "I want to be happy." The phrase "I choose joy" is more powerful.

The healing process is continual and requires acceptance at each phase. It's not a one-time event where an individual accepts their circumstance and that is it. For many chronic pain sufferers, it requires radical acceptance over and over again. Acceptance is a repeated ritual. It's not a one-time deal. It requires the act of embracing the situation or diagnosis over and over again.

The hard part of healing is we are trying to be who we used to be before the trauma or illness. That person doesn't exist anymore. The truth is we don't miss the person as much as we do the feeling.

The good news is there is a new and improved person waiting to be claimed. Claim the 2.0 version of yourself.

Here is a quote by an unknown author, "Healing is weird. Some days you're doing just fine, other days it still hurts like it's fresh. It's a process with no definitive time frame, you just have to keep going and know that when all is said and done, you're going to be okay." I often say, "Just keep on keeping on."

Long-term conditions make radical acceptance a tough pill to swallow. It's easier said than done. However, I refuse to accept that my long-term diagnosis is being in a wheelchair. I'm fighting, kicking and screaming, to find a better way. I'm scrappy and resourceful. I constantly ask myself this can't be all there is? I've researched and read thousands of comments on online support groups related to these topics.

Chronic pain patients want to spread awareness that we *"medicate to can function on most days"* rather than *"medicate to no pain or a zero"*. It's like a stop light. Red means unable to do all activities, which is considered a "bad" day. Yellow indicates being able to perform some activities with frequent breaks. Green indicates a low level of pain where many activities can be performed. Therefore, green is defined as a "good" day.

A nurse once asked me during a hospital stay what my pain relief goal was for the day and I responded with a "5". She looked at me strangely and asked what my current level was. I responded, "I am at a "9" now, hence that is why I am in this hospital. I don't expect to be a "0". In fact, I am striving for a "5" because a "5" makes life manageable. When it climbs above a "7" that is when life becomes unmanageable."

My friend reminded me that I had a limiting belief. I didn't believe that my pain would ever decrease below "5". He asked me, "What about the possibility of a "4"? This blew my mind. Since then, I have believed and experienced a "4". I just had to believe in the possibility so my mind could then make it happen.

Now back to the discussion of radical acceptance. I fight against this theory on a daily basis. Deep down my brain thinks thoughts like, "This pain will never end, and I just can't take it anymore." My heart has other plans for me. The brain and the heart rage war against each other in my body on a daily basis. It manifests itself with a non-epileptic seizure, which will be discussed in a later chapter. Literally, my body rages war against itself.

Joy is something that must be chosen daily. You and you alone must choose joy in spite of the circumstances. You must reset your mind each morning with the intention that you will find joy today no matter what.

Dig deep my friend, dig real deep. You must muster the courage to win the war over suffering on a daily basis. This book provides real and tangible methods for choosing joy over suffering.

I'm not always an optimist but I believe in the power of efficiency. There is always a better way to do something. All the options must thoroughly be explored. I want to make sure every stone is turned over. With that said, let me tell you a story about my diagnoses, trial and error process of whole body health, and wellness because healing is hard.

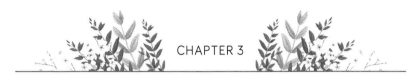

CHAPTER 3

GBS

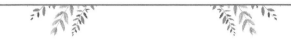

WHAT IS GUILLAIN-BARRE SYNDROME (GBS)?

*I*t was spring break in Oklahoma. The date, 3-15-14, changed my life forever. At the age of 38, I sat nervously waiting in a neurologist's office. My hands and feet were numb and tingly for the past two weeks. Walking was difficult even with a cane. My balance was poor. I was terrified to find out what was wrong with me. I already had neuropathy in my feet so this wasn't my first rodeo in a neurologist's office.

The neuropathy started in 2007 after complications from a spinal block during a c-section. I came home from the hospital with a new baby and a numb right foot. From 2007-2014, consisted of visitation with a number of specialist doctors. Thousands of dollars later and hundreds of hours wasted, I still hadn't found the answers I sought.

I turned to my husband and said, "I sure hope this new doctor knows what is wrong with me." I sat nervously fidgeting with my smart-phone. The rocking of the chair failed to calm my nerves.

I was scared of what my future held. I was sure I couldn't take much more, mentally or physically. Both my parents died a number of years prior. I was an orphan. I stopped participating in life.

My marriage was on the rocks. My son wanted a healthy mom that ran, jumped, and played with him. My faith in God and humanity was slipping through my fingers. My thoughts raced as I waited for the doctor.

Originally, my "mysterious" symptoms started two weeks prior to this neurology appointment. My primary doctor relayed that I should see a neurologist immediately. He referred me to a neurologist with a two day waiting period. This was due to the fact I had seen him once years ago so I wasn't considered a new patient.

It was the longest two days of my life. There was a three to six month waiting period to be seen by a neurologist as a new patient. This waiting period was fairly typical, no matter what part of the U.S. you lived in. Most neurologists weren't not known for their bedside manner or ease of acquiring an appointment.

My neurologist was very handsome, not quite what I expected. He had a great bedside manner and exuded compassion. He took the time to really listen. It was my experience that on average, most doctors usually allowed 10-15 minutes per patient.

This was not entirely their fault, due to the shortage of doctors and requirements from insurance companies. Most times I felt like a number and not a person during doctor visits. I was left wondering if the doctor really saw me the person, or was I viewed as an overweight diabetic that was a waste of their time.

My doctor didn't look or act like the typical doctor. He looked like a professional golfer with his polo shirt. In spite of his appearance, I had a gut feeling that this man would be my saving grace. I probably wouldn't be walking today if it weren't for him and his early detection and treatment plan. He was a game changer.

Furthermore, the neurologist that had been recommended by my chiropractor had a six month waiting period. This was a blessing in disguise because my doctor was amazing. I met the "recommended" doctor in the hospital a few days later since he was head of Neurology at the hospital.

He had a poor bedside manner and was rude to me. He suggested that maybe my pain was all in my head. He recommended I visit a psychologist, who was a partner in his practice.

He saw on my chart that I had a history of depression and anxiety. I explained to him that the numbness and tingling all over my body was not in my head but he didn't listen. He even suggested that I might not have the illness, GBS, that my doctor diagnosed me with. At this time, my doctor and he were partners in the same practice but as of 2017 they were no longer business partners.

Later, I told my doctor about my conversation with him regarding the psychologist. He smirked and said, "You are fine. You don't need to see a psychologist. I hate it when he does this. If he can't find the answer quickly from diagnostic tests, then he assumes the patient is mental." I felt relieved after he said this.

The irony is both of them were right but I didn't realize until over a year later. I often wonder if the head of neurology had actually taken the time to explain the psychological component to pain, I could have received treatment immediately. Instead, I waited over a year for a proper diagnosis of PNES. It's both a psychological and functional condition. It's classified as a movement disorder under Neurology. The confusion is it should be treated by Neurology and Psychiatry.

Furthermore, I brought a three page essay for my appointment with my doctor. It described my medical history and timeline of symptoms. I described my symptoms over the past few weeks and my prior history of neuropathy. At the urgent care clinic just two days prior, the doctor on call sent me home with pain pills and no diagnosis.

He looked up from my essay with a very worried look and said, "I think you have Guillian-Barre." I was only in his office for five minutes, when he conveyed the diagnosis.

My jaw dropped as I realized that this illness, that I can't pronounce was serious. He left the room for a few minutes. My husband and I were left with his nurse. I looked at her with a terrified glance. I asked her to spell Guillian-Barre for me. She politely wrote it on a piece of paper and handed it to me. I asked her if she knew any patients with it and she said, "No".

"Don't jump to any conclusions," my husband said. He was the eternal optimist and I was a pessimist. I highly recommend not googling your new diagnosis. Google mentioned that GBS can cause death and paralysis. I was in panic mode.

My smart phone directed me to the website, National Institute of Neurological Disorders (NIH). It defined Guillian-Barre Syndrome (also called GBS) as: "A serious autoimmune disorder where the body's immune system attacks part of the peripheral nervous system. Includes varying degrees of weakness spreading from the feet upward and can cause paralysis and can be life threatening. It is rare, afflicting only about one person in 100,000."[17]

I read the symptoms, which matched my experience. I was terrified because the website stated there was no cure. There were some treatments mentioned that help but no real cure. I read this definition out loud to my husband with a shaky voice. My husband was calm. He said, "Don't worry yet, we don't know what this means."

He conveyed that he just called a few of his colleagues to inquire if they were available to perform the Electromyography (EMG) test as soon as possible. He said a second opinion might be helpful. EMG testing is a diagnostic tool for evaluating and recording the electrical activity produced by skeletal muscles. I defined it as a torture machine. The EMG machine and I met on three prior occasions.

The EMG test assessed the health of the muscle and nerve cells that control the motor neurons. Needles were placed in all four limbs. It was a miserable experience. He explained there were two diagnostic tests that confirm a GBS diagnosis. The first was the EMG. The second was a spinal tap.

Commonly, the EMG tests for large fiber neuropathy, which is a symptom of GBS. In simple terms, large fiber neuropathy is when a limb or multiple limbs become(s) weak, tingly, numb, sore, with shooting pains. The EMG test is not a tool for diagnosing small fiber neuropathy, which is common among diabetics and chemotherapy patients.

The frustrating news is that doctors typically don't explain the importance of these tests and the difference between them. Small vs. large fiber neuropathy wasn't a common thing for patients to decipher. He explained the difference. The test results can assist with insurance companies approving additional testing, physical therapy, and orthopedic devices based on the diagnosis. GBS presents with abnormal muscle and nerve readings on the EMG test.

The following morning, I limped into his office using a cane. I climbed onto the hard and freezing exam table. He inserted large needles in all four limbs. During this procedure, I explained that I had had the EMG test on prior occasions and the results were normal. The test took about an hour. My doctor and his nurse were awesome. They re-arranged their schedule so they could complete my EMG test right away.

The story of my chronic pain journey from a physical stand-point began in 2007. However, I had suffered from on and off again back and hip pain since the age of seventeen. I had been rear-ended driving home from school.

The mental aspect started when I was eight, 1988. Severe pain was my constant companion for seven years since my c-section and birth of my only child. I referred to my son as my ten pound preemie, since he entered the world at ten pounds and two weeks early. Currently, at the age of 12 is 6'1 with a men's size 12 shoe.

The anesthesiologist was late and my OB GYN and nurse were waiting on him. It seemed like the spinal block was rushed. After he inserted the needle in my spine, I felt something was wrong. My legs began to shake and tremor. I wondered if this feeling was normal but before I could ask, my doctor began the c-section procedure. Then, chaos ensued.

My right foot remained numb and tingly after the spinal block when the pain meds wore off. On the second day after my c-section, I tried to walk from the bathroom to my bed when my back locked up. It was the most intense pain. I could not move. My husband and the nurse carried me to the bed.

I left the hospital with a limp two days later. My right foot was numb and the pain was intense. I referred to this moment as the beginning of the end. I was never the same after this. My health gradually deteriorated, both physically and mentally.

Thus, I continued my history of neuropathy discussion. A few weeks after my c-section in 2007, x-rays showed I had a herniated disc in my lower back. I began physical therapy but it didn't help. In hindsight, I didn't work on the assigned PT exercises like I should have.

I even had spinal injections. They also didn't help. I also went to a chiropractor, which helped in the short term but was expensive. Acupuncture also helped in the short term.

The medical decision I regretted the most was back surgery. My regrets were: that I didn't exercise daily such as walking or swimming and my lack of weight loss. A year after my son was born, I had an L4-S1 spinal fusion. I still have the metal hardware in my back as of

2020. My hope was that it would decrease my foot, back, and hip pain, but that was not the case.

The decision to have back surgery was a short term solution. Typically, I had heard that people who have one back surgery, another one would be required some day. This was because the section above the surgery site weakens over time. I experienced this phenomenon about eight years after the fusion surgery.

> In the U.S., we seek quick fix solutions. We want an easy solution that doesn't require much effort. So many surgeries in the U.S., mine included, are unnecessarily performed. Therefore, I implore those considering back surgery, not to do it unless walking is no longer possible. I also advise getting a second opinion. In some cases, a third or fourth might be necessary. These decisions will affect the rest of your life so take the time to consider wisely.

Subsequently, I bit my lip as phase II of the EMG continued, which was the most painful part of the test. The machine sent shocks through my limbs that made me want to scream. Tears rolled down my face as my body jerked and twitched. I told him that the foot pain reached it's worse level about two weeks ago.

Next, I conveyed my experience with a local rheumatologist. He diagnosed me with Fibromyalgia around 2009. He prescribed a medication, called Savella. It's an serotonin-norepinephrine reuptake inhibitor (SNRI) that is prescribed for fibromyalgia.

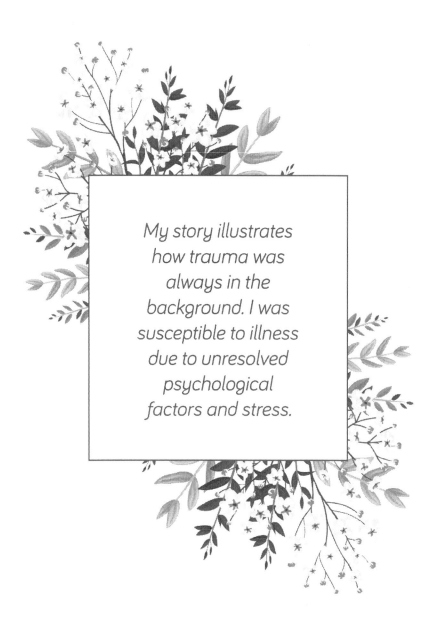

My story illustrates how trauma was always in the background. I was susceptible to illness due to unresolved psychological factors and stress.

Savella helped but the side effect was excessive sweating. I took Savella for about a year then quit during the summertime, when the sweating was exasperated. In hindsight, some of the sweating could have been attributed to anxiety. I didn't get sweaty palms but rather full body sweating.

The rheumatologist also suggested I go on an all plant based diet. However, I refused and kept eating the same old way. I clearly had not learned my lesson.

My primary doctor then prescribed Talwin, which was a mild opiate. Talwin managed the pain for a few years. It was not a widely prescribed medication so it was hard to locate a pharmacy that supplied it.

He saw the frustration and pain on my face as I continued my medical history. I said, "Honestly, when most doctors see that I am diabetic and overweight, they write me off and stop looking for anything else. They tell me that 100% of my foot numbness was due to diabetes."

I explained to them that I was a Type II diabetic. I had only been diabetic for six months since it started during pregnancy. I said, "My blood sugar wasn't even that high, 120-140. The normal range was around 80 to 100. That was not high enough to cause the severe numbness in the right foot."

Many doctors over the years conveyed, "It must be from pre-diabetes," and I responded, "I think it was from the spinal block." Some doctors agreed that the pain was caused by the spinal block. However, most believed that it was from diabetes. I have had several neurologists tell me that pre-diabetes can cause neuropathy.

And yet, I continued to rattle on about my story during the long EMG test. I was so grateful that a doctor was actually listening and letting me talk. He was very funny and the talking helped to keep my mind off the pain. I explained the last two weeks in detail.

It started when I noticed the numbness in my feet was worse. My first thought was that the neuropathy was getting worse. A week after the initial onset, I remembered waking up one morning and my hands were numb.

At first, I just thought that I had slept on them wrong. A few hours later, the numbness in my hands continued as it spread up my arms. I went to work thinking it would go away. I left work early and went to urgent care. The doctor had no clue what was wrong with me. He spent one minute with me, gave me some pain pills, and sent me home.

That aside, I continued with my hour long story about how the pain began to spread upward into my thighs, arms, & face. I was terrified. The pain was equal on both sides. My balance was poor, walking became difficult, and my blood pressure was all over the place. I had trouble breathing.

He explained that my EMG test only showed minor abnormalities of large fiber neuropathy. However, given my symptoms, he still felt like GBS was the correct diagnosis. He ordered some additional testing and labs to be done at the hospital.

He felt that I should be admitted to the hospital that day. He said it was important for me to wear a heart monitor and oxygen. His nurse organized all my hospital admittance papers and reserved a hospital bed. I was amazed at how fast this process was happening. Their admittance process was like a well-oiled machine. They were a true doctor and nurse team.

Furthermore, my doctor came that evening to visit me and came five out of the six days that I was in the hospital. I thanked him for re-arranging his schedule for me. He told me, "Patients like you are the reason I became a doctor." I cried as I felt overcome with human kindness and compassion. I told him there weren't many doctors like him. He humbly smiled.

Next, he explained that I needed to have a spinal tap to evaluate the protein in the spinal fluid. He said, "If the protein level is elevated then that confirms the GBS diagnosis." He also ordered an MRI to rule out MS (multiple sclerosis). The scans were normal.

The spinal tap was very painful and scary. The thought of a huge needle in my spine was terrifying, especially after what happened with the spinal block during my c-section. This was why he ordered it to be done under X-ray to reduce the risk.

The spinal tap is also called lumbar puncture and is used to evaluate the cerebrospinal fluid. The spinal tap is a standard test that is typically used when neurological symptoms of numbness and tingling are present.

"The cerebrospinal fluid (CSF) that bathes the spinal cord and brain contains more protein than usual in Guillain-Barré syndrome but has a normal CSF cell count. Therefore, a spinal tap (a procedure in which the doctor inserts a needle into the patient's lower back to draw cerebrospinal fluid from the spinal column) may need to be performed. The peripheral white blood cell count in Guillain-Barré syndrome is normal."[17] My results revealed only a minor elevation of protein in the spinal fluid.

He explained that he still felt that I had GBS in spite of these results. He explained that there was no cure but there were two types of treatment that could help. The main clue to the diagnosis was the ascending pain that was equal on both sides. There were no other known neurological diseases with this symptom.

One was called IVIG (Intravenous Immunoglobulin) and the other was called plasmapheresis. He explained that the IVIG treatment was more effective for GBS cases in his opinion. IVIG is defined by the NIH, "A blood product prepared from the serum of between 1000 and 15,000 blood donors per batch. It is the treatment of choice for patients with antibody deficiencies."[17]

Subsequently, he ordered five days of IVIG. It is defined by the company KabaFusion as, "A process that provides healthy antibodies to block the immune and inflammatory processes and bind rogue autoantibodies and remove them from circulation. It was donated plasma that was filtered and administered very slowly via IV. It replaced the "bad" cells with those of "healthy" donors."[18]

The process took five hours to administer and can cause bad headaches. He told the nurses to administer very slowly and not rush it because of the headache side effect. Thanks to him, I had no headaches.

The hardest part of the treatment was that the nurses lacked knowledge about what size needles to use. IVIG is a thick liquid and requires a larger needle. The nurse used a smaller needle and it backed up in my arm which was quite painful.

> IVIG was very expensive and costs around $8,000/day in the U.S.

I was so blessed to have had amazing insurance that covered 100% of the bill. My insurance never even questioned covering it. I had heard stories of insurance companies denying coverage for it. Also, IVIG can be administered at home if insurance approves it. Protocol is every 22-30 days as ordered by a doctor. Patients that acquire the chronic form of GBS, called chronic inflammatory demyelinating polyneuropath (CIDP) usually get this treatment monthly.

I met my out of pocket maximum during this hospital stay, which meant my healthcare would cost $0 for the rest of the year. Plasmapheresis treatments are often given to patients with auto-immune diseases. It's more cost effective than IVIG.

Plasmapheresis defined by the Healthline Media is, "A process where the liquid or plasma in the blood is separated from the cells with a machine. In ill patients, plasma can contain antibodies that attack the immune system."[19] Neurologists differ on which treatment is more effective.

Physical and occupational therapy nurses visited every day while I was in the hospital. The therapists would tie a belt around me and hold on to me as we walked the halls with the aid of a walker. When I was alone in my room, I would use a wheelchair to go to the bathroom. I was so scared of falling. My balance was poor. I was afraid I was going to face plant on the bathroom floor.

The occupational therapist would have me perform hand exercises. I would practice buttoning shirts that were glued to a wood block. They had a web mesh device that looked like a spider web. They showed me how to use it to strengthen my hands and fingers and recommended that I buy one when I get home from the hospital.

This device is called Power Web (hand exerciser), and can be purchased on Amazon. It's also helpful for arthritis patients to improve dexterity. This began my five year journey of physical therapy off and on.

The IVIG treatment made me very sleepy so I slept all day and watched my iPad at night. I binge watched the entire series of "Veronica Mars" in the hospital. Thus, began my addiction to Netflix and binge watching entire seasons of t.v. shows. "Veronica Mars" was a great distraction. While I was lying in a hospital bed in Tulsa Oklahoma, my husband and son went to New York without me.

It was spring break and I was excited about going to New York for the first time. However, God had other plans for me. Exactly five years later, God provided a way for me to visit New York and be part of the "This is Pain" (www.thisispain.com) marketing campaign, sponsored by the ACPA to bring awareness to chronic pain. My story is featured there.

The NYC trip gave me my confidence back. I was terrified to walk the crowded NYC streets because I used a cane. I was afraid I couldn't keep up. I used a cane in my right hand and held on to my husband's arm with the left. My husband waited to tell me until the end of the night that I had walked six miles in one day. Of course I had to take many breaks and a nap in between but I did it! Hallelujah! God is good!

&

Nevertheless, I knew that my symptoms were less severe than the typical ones listed on the internet for GBS. The internet mentioned every GBS case was unique. I was blessed to only have a mild version of it. Also, there are several variants of GBS. They are: Acute inflammatory demyelinating polyradiculoneuropathy (AIDP), the most widely recognized form of GBS in Western countries. The variants known as acute motor axonal neuropathy (AMAN) and acute motor-sensory axonal neuropathy (AMSAN), and Miller-Fisher syndrome are well recognized.

My "mild" case was due to my doctor's excellent care and early detection. My hospital stay was only six days. Many GBS patients stay in some form of hospital or rehab facility for months or even years. Many patients are on ventilators and feeding tubes. I left the hospital using a cane. However, I also used a wheelchair or rolling walker with a seat for anything that required a lot of walking. This is also true for my present day activity in 2020. The rolling walker with a basket underneath and a cup holder is a lifesaver when going to festivals or concerts.

In addition, the literature on GBS was limited. Most books described severe cases. Also, I haven't found any books or resources that explained how severe the "residual effects" associated with GBS are. Most of my knowledge about residuals came from watching YouTube videos from other GBS warriors (#gbswarrior).

Also, in my research I had trouble finding info on the long term recovery process. Most of the books were focused on the acute part of the disease and managing the emergency related symptoms. I wish I had known how difficult it was and all the ups and downs related to recovery.

I published some YouTube videos about GBS residuals and recovery on my social media handle (@chronicpainhacker) as well as other videos on life hacks for dealing with chronic pain.

There weren't any books that described the milder cases of GBS. It was important to note that these "milder" cases wreaked havoc on the lives of many patients and their loved ones. The "milder" cases required the patient to fight harder for answers because their symptoms weren't as textbook or obvious. However, the "milder" symptoms could lead to dire circumstances if ignored. A fall caused by weakness associated with GBS, could cause life threatening complications.

> The cause of GBS is unknown. However, there are many stressors that contribute to the immune system going haywire.

There has been some speculation that it can be caused by flu shots. My doctor told me not to get the flu shot ever again. I know of two cases in Texas that were caused by the flu shot. Many doctors are suggesting that patients use the flu mist instead of the shot. I am scared for my family and friends to get flu shots.

Other speculated causes are: respiratory viruses, Zika virus from mosquitoes, surgery, childbirth, extreme stress, or a weakened immune system. Also, it has been speculated that Native Americans are more susceptible to GBS. I am Native American of Delaware and Cherokee descent. In my case, I had all the risk factors listed above except for Zika.

In retrospect, I remembered that my co-workers were sick with a respiratory virus and then I became ill. A week later, the GBS symptoms started. I was still recovering from a complicated hernia surgery so my immune system was shot. I had eight surgeries in about seven years so my body had enough. I was physically and emotionally drained.

My story illustrates how trauma was always in the background. I was susceptible to illness due to unresolved psychological factors and big life stressors. For example, I had four relatives pass away in four months from January through April 2014. I was emotionally spent.

I think GBS is more prevalent than we realize. It gets mis-di-agnosed easily in the United States, and even more in third-world countries, where access to doctors and medicine is limited. For example, when the symptoms first started, I went to urgent care. The doctors didn't have a clue and sent me home with pain pills. Doctors treat the tip of the iceberg.

It's reported that the odds of contracting GBS are 1/100,000. Many doctors don't take the time to listen fully or they are so over-booked with patients, that they don't order any diagnostic tests. Many patients go to the ER or urgent care in pain and are sent home with pain pills, no follow up plan, and no diagnostic tests performed. Part of this is because of the long wait time to see a neurologist at his/her regular office.

Paralysis can set in quickly and require an immediate hospital admittance and many cases an ICU admission. The other extreme is a milder paralysis as with my case that feels more like severe neuropathy and is more difficult to diagnose. Unless the patient tells the doctor that the pain is ascending and equal on both sides, it is hard to distinguish GBS from other diseases like multiple sclerosis (MS) or Lyme disease. My personal opinion is that it is more like fifty persons in 100,000.

The NIH, "Reports about 20,000 U.S. cases per year that can affect any age. In 2016, the news reported several GBS cases in South America and in Florida due to the Zika virus. Both sexes are equally prone to the disorder. The syndrome is rare; however, afflicting only about one person in 100,000 worldwide. Children, who rarely develop Guillain-Barre syndrome, generally recover more completely than adults.[17]

According to The Mayo Clinic, "Among adults recovering from Guillain-Barre syndrome:

- About 80 percent can walk independently six months after diagnosis

- About 60 percent fully recover motor strength one year after diagnosis

- About 5 to 10 percent have very delayed and incomplete recovery

The recovery period may be as little as a few weeks or as long as a few years. About thirty percent of those with Guillain-Barré still have a residual weakness after three years. About three percent of patients may suffer a relapse of muscle weakness and tingling sensations many years after the initial attack."[20]

GBS patients face not only physical difficulties, but emotionally painful periods as well. It's often extremely difficult for patients to adjust to sudden paralysis and dependence on others for help with routine daily activities. Patients sometimes need psychological counseling to help them adapt. I certainly took for granted the ability to walk, run, or even comb my hair.

Scientists are concentrating on finding new treatments and refining existing ones. They are also looking at the workings of the immune system to find which cells are responsible for beginning and carrying out the attack on the nervous system.

> The fact that so many cases of GBS begin after a viral or bacterial infection, suggest that certain characteristics of some viruses and bacteria may activate the immune system inappropriately.

According to The NIH, "Investigators are searching for those characteristics. Certain proteins or peptides in viruses and bacteria may be the same as those found in myelin, and the generation of antibodies to neutralize the invading viruses or bacteria could trigger the attack on the myelin sheath. As noted previously, neurological scientists, immunologists, virologists, and pharmacologists are all working collaboratively to learn how to prevent this disorder and to make better therapies available when it strikes."[17]

Also, there is a great support organization, GBS/CIDP Foundation International, which provides website, seminars, phone support, walk and roll marathons, and newsletters to GBS and CIDP patients.

I attended their annual international symposium in San Antonio in 2016. Each year it's located in a different U.S. or Canadian city. Many doctors and health professionals spoke about GBS/CIDP. We broke into small groups with other patients. Meeting other patients and sharing symptoms was the most beneficial part of this seminar.

Furthermore, I met patients that were one year to eleven years since diagnosis. We discovered we were all still dealing with the same recovery issues, known as residuals in the medical community. The most common was the weak ankle reflexes, which made falls more prevalent. We all told our tales of how we think we contracted GBS.

A thirty-something woman, who contracted GBS during pregnancy, was still able to deliver a healthy baby. However, she suffered from many of the same physical symptoms as everyone at the table of my small group. The people in my group that seemed to recover faster, were much younger at the time of on-set.

Also, I met a very nice man from California, who was eleven years out and not much better off than I was at the two year mark. This didn't give me hope about my long-term physical outlook but it helped to know I wasn't alone. I left the seminar feeling deflated.

Finally, we discussed how other pre-existing health conditions or age prior to the GBS onset, impacted one's recovery. The quality of experienced physical and occupational therapists played a huge role. For example, conditions like diabetes, surgeries, back problems, auto-immune diseases, fibromyalgia, and neuropathy played a big role in the ability to recover from GBS faster.

My prior failed back surgery, diagnosed depression and anxiety, and diabetic neuropathy in my limbs, fibromyalgia, and non-epileptic seizures made my recovery more difficult. Many health care professionals were confused about my diagnosis and recovery. I think they were looking for just one area to focus on instead of looking at the whole body. I was a hot mess and they didn't know where to start.

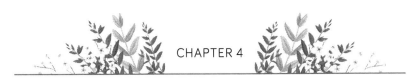

CHAPTER 4

NON-EPILEPTIC SEIZURES (PNES)

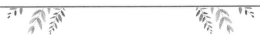

*T*he year was 2015. I was diagnosed with a rare neurological movement disorder. The disorder is referred to as psychogenic seizures, nonepileptic attack disorder (NEADS), conversion disorder, or psychogenic non-epileptic seizures (PNES). They are also referred to as "pseudo seizures". They are referred to as NEADS in Europe.

These are non-epileptic episodes that are often misdiagnosed as epilepsy. There is limited research or books about PNES so diagnosis is a difficult road for many. The many acronyms for this diagnosis causes confusion among doctors and patients.

I fought the PNES diagnosis with every fiber of my being. I wanted my diagnosis to be solely based on physical symptoms. I didn't want to believe that my mind was making me sick. I knew I had some anxiety and depression but I had no idea the severity. This was because PNES caused a dissociative state, which caused me to "zone out" frequently.

Depression is like a small crack in a dam that slowly expands over time until one day it bursts. Oftentimes, people are caught off guard when the dam breaks and they wonder if they were more depressed than they realized.

The stress of having GBS was the straw that broke the camel's back. My mind and body had been through so much at this point. The paralysis brought upon from GBS, resulted in having to learn to walk again. The stress of my "new normal" was overwhelming. I was in mourning for the person I used to be.

I began an intense inpatient and outpatient physical therapy program that lasted on and off for five years. Thankfully, the exercises can be performed at home. They are still part of my daily exercise regimen.

My PT (physical therapist) taught me how to walk with proper posture, how to get up from a seated position, how to sleep effectively with pillows and positioning, and how to drive with pillows. We worked on my posture at great lengths as well as lifestyle modifications. I was surprised how much a wedge pillow can help position weak muscles.

On many occasions, I left the PT clinic in tears. I felt like I would never be able to do the exercises she recommended. She was amazing. The problem was my belief that I couldn't get better. In my case, belief was the entire battle, no half way about it.

The pain I felt after completing the exercises was intense, leaving me weak. I often had to take a nap after exercising because of the overwhelming fatigue I felt. My muscles felt like jello. Movement was vital but so difficult. I fought for every step I took. The infamous catch-22, damned if you do and damned if you don't, characterized my life. Muscles atrophy quicker than people realize, making constant movement vital.

I grieved some devastating physical losses with falls, mobility limitations, and failed surgeries. The past five years (2014-2019), were characterized by bouncing back and forth between walking unassisted with a limp. I also used a cane, walker, and wheelchair depending on how I felt or if an event required a long walk. These were the worst years of my life. I feel like I lost the entire year of 2014. As of 2020, I no longer consider it a waste because it allowed a journey of awakening to bubble within my soul.

Managing fatigue was the hardest thing for me to tackle. Fatigue was harder to deal with than the pain. Many times, I simply didn't have the energy required to complete basic tasks like: exercising, cooking, shopping, walking, and showering. I used most of my energy on remaining upright after numerous falls. Also, seizures cause severe fatigue.

The first quarter of 2020, I felt like I was finally practicing radical acceptance on a consistent basis. I choose joy daily sometimes successfully and other times not. It took five years to create and implement this process. The following chapters describe my experience with healing.

MANAGING THIS DIAGNOSIS

My anxiety was and is crippling, literally. I write this paragraph in both present and past tense because it's a life-long condition that needs to be managed. Typically, after a PNES seizure, depending on the intensity, walking aids like a cane or rolling walker, are and were needed. The seizures weaken (ed) my entire body making it hard to recover. On many occasions, they wipe (d) me out for hours or even an entire day.

Every single step was shaky. I felt like I dragged twenty pound sandbags behind me. It was very hard to gain momentum. I repeated this mantra, "Power through, power through…just a few more steps."

Furthermore, the effect of chronically ill persons can be devastating on family dynamics. Everyone involved is overwhelmed as new family members take on tasks that were previously handled by the ill person. Supportive friends and family make all the difference in the world.

At times, I felt guilty that my son had to assist me so much. I tried to focus on the idea that he learned important life skills. He learned at a young age, responsibility. He cooked, cleaned, and washed laundry, which were valuable skills to have.

The extra effort that my son and husband put forth was not lost on me. They definitely stepped up to the plate and took over the household on days that I couldn't get out of bed. Family members can be overwhelmed in the beginning with this new added responsibility. That was where professional support groups came in. I can't recommend enough, the value of support groups. They were helpful for the entire family.

For example, my husband attended an intensive three week chronic pain rehabilitation support group program with me in Ohio at the Cleveland Clinic. The spouses and family members were able to ask questions of the doctors. They listened in our group sessions. This was valuable information for my husband. As a result of this trip, I was better able to participate in life. I had checked out of life and had no desire to press on.

The rehab program combined physical and occupational therapy as well as individual and group talk therapy. The therapists instructed us on how to perform household chores with proper posture to prevent injury and further pain. They even taught us how to get in and out of a bathtub safely. I still use this technique.

One of the doctors said something I will never forget, "When you just introduced yourself to the group, you described yourself as a patient and not a person." Up to that point, I didn't realize I was letting my diagnosis be my identity. The light bulb came on and sparked the journey to find out who I really am.

This path led to facilitating my own chronic pain support group in Austin, Texas. I trained as a meeting facilitator sponsored by the "American Chronic Pain Association" (ACPA). They are a non for profit company that provides free sources and information, see website link in the resources section of this book.

The founder of the ACPA had attended this rehabilitation program years before me and thus formed the ACPA in 1980. They have devoted 40 years of support and education in pain management skills to people with pain, family, friends, and health care professionals.

The next essential thing that happened at the Cleveland Clinic, was that I met the first neurologist to diagnose me with PNES. He called them "pseudo seizures" that start in the musculoskeletal system as opposed to the brain. He verified this via an electroencephalogram (EEG) which lasted five minutes. I immediately thought that the word "pseudo" meant he thought I was faking them.

During this test, the technician simulated the environment with flashing lights. I began seizing on the exam table. I was sure it was a real seizure. I was so confused when the results confirmed PNES over epilepsy. Once I arrived back in Texas, I began to get second opinions from other neurologists.

PNES seizures were devastating. They wrecked my whole world. Also, the reaction of others added to the devastation. I once had a neurologist just stare at me during an episode in his presence and he said nothing. He was very rude. I guess he felt I was a waste of his time since he wanted to handle a real epilepsy case.

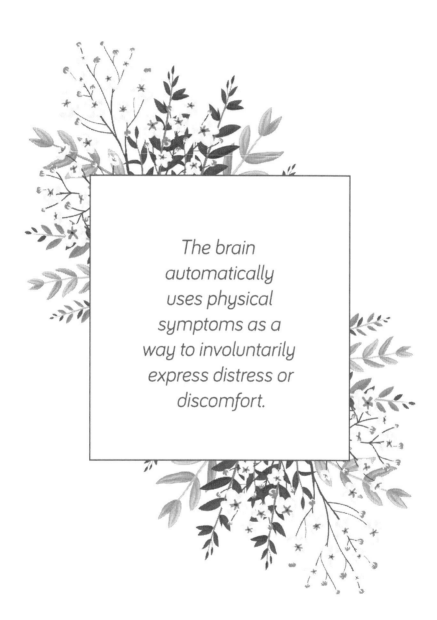

The brain automatically uses physical symptoms as a way to involuntarily express distress or discomfort.

Ironically, PNES was and is considered a neurological move-ment disorder. Another neurologist repeated the same offense. He seemed upset, when he couldn't find what he thought was a real neurological condition. He sent me for several unneeded tests.

Many people have never heard of PNES. I certainly never had. They are not aware of the distressing factors that can be associated with PNES. I was that person. I would say, "I am not that stressed."

Depression caused me not to recognize the amount of stress I was under. I saw a movie about hysterical blindness as a kid but never believed it was real until now. For example, the musician, Ray Charles, experienced hysterical blindness due to a childhood trauma. His sight never returned.

PNES came with denial of distress recently or otherwise. The site, www.nonepileptic seizures.com, is a great resource for FAQs and a list of doctors that specialize.

The brain automatically uses physical symptoms as a way to involuntarily express distress or discomfort. These automatic brain responses may develop due to an accumulation of stressful factors and or learned behaviors, or troubling experiences over time. However, people don't always feel distressed or upset right before a PNES episode. They might not recall any major distress months or years before the onset of PNES.

I absolutely feel distressed right before an episode. Also, too much activity without rest in between caused episodes. According to www.nonepileptic seizures.com, "PNES is a response to stimuli not entering conscious awareness in the same way as one may step out of the way of a puddle while walking and talking to someone without ever becoming aware of the puddle".[21]

Seizures surfaced after I was exposed to bright light, flashing light, or loud noises. Police and ambulance lights were difficult to look at. I've learned to wear earplugs and tinted glasses. My doctor suggested noise canceling headphones.

Also, avoidance of overhead lights was helpful. Opting for softer lighting was beneficial, such as lamps placed behind me. Fluorescent lighting found in many commercial establishments bothered me as well. Infrared heat lamps soothed my distressed muscles.

My right eye started to twitch when the stimuli response was too much for me to handle. This was the first hint that a PNES seizure was on the way. Eye twitching is a common response to stress.

The cumulative effect of thirty-five years of unresolved stress, anxiety, and PTSD, presented itself as PNES seizures in my body. My body converted mental anguish into physical pain. They caused intense pain, moans and screams (vocal spasms), twitching, convulsing, muscle spasms, paralyzation, and fatigue.

My body betrayed me daily, even in my sleep. I woke up with a twisted, rotated feeling in my back and rib cage that was quite painful. Often, I woke up feeling like I was dragged behind a car in my sleep. There were a few occasions where I woke up on my nightstand due to convulsions. This required pillows to be placed between myself and the nightstand. A body pillow provided some stability.

Another symptom of anxiety is teeth grinding. My grinding at night was so severe that I cracked a tooth even with my retainer on. I also wore the enamel off my bottom front teeth. I had to get a special heavy duty night guard. My mother also suffered from teeth grinding.

My right side was significantly weaker than my left because my left side isn't affected during the seizures. It is common for only one side of the body to be affected with PNES. I had trouble lifting my right arm.

Sometimes, I looked down at myself while seated and noticed that my right side was slouching, due to the painful rotation in my back around the L3 region (spinal position in the middle of the lumbar spine). My prior lumbar fusion surgery complicated this matter.

Luckily, my PT had taught my family how to un-rotate my back which was a lifesaver. It definitely saved time and money on chiropractic and PT visits. She also told me to use pillows to prop myself up so I can remain in alignment for longer periods of time after spinal manipulation. Every single day my back rotated and I had to reset it. This was especially true after exercising, prolonged standing, bending, or carrying something heavy. Currently, this process still needs to be completed daily.

I had pillows everywhere; in the car, on the couch, and my bed. I slept with five pillows. I had a small pillow and yoga block that I took with me everywhere. I placed it behind my back to keep from slouching. A yoga block was used to prop up my feet while seated in a chair. It helped take the pressure off my back.

Comfortable seating was crucial. I liked to sit in padded booths at restaurants because wood and metal chairs were very uncomfortable. I sometimes avoided places with uncomfortable seating.

Coordination was difficult because my left and right side failed to sync up. It also made typing or holding things difficult. I broke many dishes and spilled something at least once daily. For example, I can't tell how much pressure to apply to objects such as, the pressure required to type on my phone or laptop because of the numbness and tingling in my hands. Voice to text applications have been a lifesaver.

The neuropathy in my hands caused me to spill coffee on my work laptop after being hospitalized with GBS. I fried it. I gave my notice to my employer shortly after this happened. I felt I couldn't work anymore, not only from physical symptoms but from the intense brain fog. I couldn't focus and my memory loss caused significant delays in job duty performance.

My anxiety level also increased making a stressful job feel impossible. The walk to the bathroom and to the community printer at my work office was too much for me. It required too much energy.

Not to mention, I had to park three blocks away. There was no handicap parking and a shortage of parking period. I had amazing coworkers that would pick me up and take me to the door as well as food and drink deliveries. Working from home was an option, but was too difficult due to the brain fog and fatigue. I could not hold my head up.

Next, twitching was a very common symptom of PNES. I had a friend with PNES that twitched in both eyes in rapid movement. Also, the muscles became very stiff, which caused a "Frankenstein" kind of walk. My gait was characterized by short, jerky steps.

Even on good days, walking was still a challenge. I felt very frustrated that I couldn't take walks with my family. Therefore, yoga was helpful because a good workout could be obtained without having to walk, jump, or run. Swimming in a heated pool was also beneficial.

The seizures were so intense that the muscles became weak and tingly, making everything difficult. Muscle relaxers helped but not as much as I had hoped. Thankfully, after a few hours, the muscles strengthened enough to walk with a limp. Improvement of symptoms typically came within four hours of the seizure.

However, on bad days they seemed to ruin my entire day. Long naps were required for recovery. Depression also played a big role in this. Depression locked me into a "stuck" position. Depression looks like sleeping too much, lack of hygiene, and sitting for extended periods.

Sometimes, I used a walker or cane after the seizures. If I used the techniques discussed in the following chapters, my day would definitely have a different outcome. I walked unassisted for short distances but still had trouble with distance walking. Currently, I often take my walker to events that require lots of walking or standing.

I didn't let it stop me from attending concerts. Many of them attended in a wheelchair or rolling walker with a seat. I was surprised at how organized the American Disabilities Act (ADA) was at various music venues around Austin. One venue gave me a very important person (VIP) seat with balcony access when they saw me with my walker.

꒰꒱

Furthermore, my frustration level increased when trying to explain to people that this kind of fatigue was no joke. It wasn't the same as being really tired. This is a serious medical condition and patients aren't faking this.

The need to explain myself to others was important as I didn't want people to think I was lazy. My therapist told me not to waste my breath trying to convince folks because they wouldn't get it. Currently, I no longer care what others think regarding this matter.

Energy levels were greatly affected so I had to take a break after each activity. Pacing oneself was critical and required trial and error. This took years to accomplish the balance between "too much" and "too little." The struggle was and is real.

Spoon theory is a metaphor in the chronic illness community. It describes the amount of energy both mental and physical required to complete a task. Spoons are a visual representation for a unit of energy. Each activity requires a certain amount of spoons. Once the spoon is used, it can't be replenished until rest is achieved.

It's the process used to ration the number of spoons used in a given day. The theory also seeks to improve empathy among the healthy community. Awareness of what it's like to complete tasks when facing chronic pain on a daily basis. Healthy individuals have an unlimited supply of spoons compared to "spoonies" who only have a certain number to last the entire day. The term spoonie indicates persons with chronic physical and mental conditions. This term is widely used on social media.

PNES VS. EPILEPSY DIAGNOSIS

My most asked question about PNES is: "How do you tell the difference between a PNES seizure and epilepsy?" The diagnostic testing tool is a video EEG. It records the electrical activity of the brain. Most neurologists order a seventy-two hour video test to be completed at home to give them better data.

Doctors are more confident in the diagnosis if seventy-two hours of video recording can be reviewed by a neurologist. Electrodes are placed all over the scalp. Then, they are connected to the EEG machine. A video recorder is also used even during sleep to see if episodes occur at night.

My seventy-two hour results revealed numerous episodes per day/night, resulting in a diagnosis of PNES. No wonder I woke up feeling tired. Finally, I had three doctor's opinions that I definitely had PNES.

It can also be helpful to record PNES episodes on smartphones to show to your neurologist. It's reasonable for additional tests to be ordered (MRI or CT scan) to rule out other possibilities, such as other neurological conditions. This is just another step to confirm the diagnosis of PNES.

Some neurologists will immediately refer a PNES patient to psychiatry, and tell them they don't need to be seen further by neurology. This happened to me. I got bounced back and forth between neurology and psychiatry. It was frustrating for everyone. In my opinion, a patient needs to be seen by both specialities. Currently, I see both every six months.

Currently, I visit my neurologist every six months since acquiring GBS in 2014. However, I visited several neurologists that weren't helpful before I met my current neurologist. She has a great bedside manner, which is rare for neurologists in my opinion. Compassionate medical care is essential in managing PNES. Patients are already anxious, and doctors stating, "It's all in your head, your faking, and I can't help you" isn't helpful.

Unfortunately, some doctors, friends, and family think the person is faking the seizures. Many doctors and nurses are not well-trained in PNES, so the patient is treated like they are crazy.

There are other conditions that also cause a physical response to emotional difficulties such as: IBS (Irritable Bowel Syndrome), panic attacks, fibromyalgia, double vision, blurred vision, chronic fatigue, and tension headaches. Yes, I have all these conditions. They often accompany each other as a package deal. As if just one diagnosis isn't enough.

The number of people affected with PNES is not exactly known due to misdiagnosis and lack of understanding from medical staff. The PNES site explains that, "Out of ten patients seen in an epilepsy inpatient unit for difficult to treat seizures, two out of five actually have a diagnosis of PNES."[21] This site also has a list of mental health doctors that specialize in PNES in the U.S. and Canada.

Studies have shown there is no effective medication to cure PNES. However, medications may be recommended to treat other disorders that frequently occur in patients with PNES. Anti epileptic drugs and benzodiazepines are often prescribed. It's my opinion that these make PNES symptoms worse.

I had unpleasant experiences with these and couldn't handle the side effects of extreme brain fog. This is why I prefer the drug Vistaril because it's safer for long term use. It's in the antihistamine family. My psychiatrist doesn't like to prescribe benzodiazepines due to the side effect of dementia and risk for addiction after long time use.

The recommended treatment is: psychiatry, talk therapy, acupuncture, yoga, mindfulness, meditation, lifestyle changes, CBT, DBT, EMDR, stress reducing techniques, cannabis, and alternative living options discussed in the following chapters.

Cessation of PNES episodes or significant reduction in the frequency, has been reported in over half of the cases using any of the above mentioned techniques. I have found meditation and CBD to be the most effective for me.

It's possible to be diagnosed with PNES and epilepsy as well as other neurological conditions. PNES also states that, "Approximately ten to twenty-five percent of adults with PNES and up to twenty-five percent of children with PNES also have epilepsy."[21] I have an online contact that has cerebral palsy and both types of seizures.

The lack of support and generally poor attitude from medical professionals caused me to seek out compassionate doctors and therapists. For online support via Facebook, check out the group, "Psychogenic Non-Epileptic Seizures." Read the comments from others' posts and learn some new management techniques as well as gain support from a community of people dealing with PNES. You are not alone. It will be ok. It's possible to get your life back but it requires dedication and commitment on a regular basis.

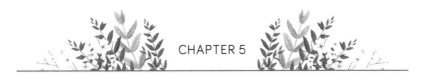

CHAPTER 5

PTSD

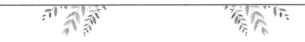

I had met several women online and in person that suffered from PNES. I discussed with my current neurologist that PNES seemed to affect women more than men. Also, women who had unresolved trauma, neglect, natural disasters, accidents, sudden loss of loved one, significant medical issues, caring for ailing parent, sexual abuse, and PTSD, were more likely to experience PNES.

I experienced all of these over a span of 38 years. She agreed with these comments. "Approximately, fifty percent of patients with PNES carry a diagnosis of PTSD," according to the nonepileptic seizure website."[21]

Many questions arrived in my inbox asking how to tell the difference between epilepsy and PNES seizures. My doctor explained the difference between the two categories of seizures. Also, she conveyed that most of her PNES patients were in wheelchairs. She complimented my approach to my diagnosis and explained I was doing all the right things to manage my illness.

"Presentation is different, where with PNES, it typically affects one side of the body. Epilepsy typically involves both sides of the body. Duration of the seizure is different. Typically, epileptic seizures are quicker from one minute up to twenty minutes. Whereas, PNES seizures are much longer and can go on for twenty four hours.

"PNES is characterized more by muscle twitches and spasms. Epilepsy is more a jerking motion that can be very intense. There is no loss of consciousness with PNES. However, it can be dangerous because walking during a PNES seizure could cause a fall according to the nonepileptic seizure website."[21]

The chapters below discuss alternative options and tools to help manage the diagnosis of PNES. One of those tools, eye movement desensitization and reprocessing (EMDR), helped to resolve my PTSD from childhood trauma.

Relief from PNES can be achieved, but mental health must be maintained on a regular basis. On days that I skipped my meditation or there was high humidity and or barometric pressure changes, I noticed my right eye twitching and seizures were quick to follow.

Sometimes, the seizure could be stopped even after twitching had begun but it required meditating in a dark, quiet space. PTSD is not only experienced by war veterans but by many people experiencing the kinds of trauma listed above.

Fast forward to the present, 2020, I am happy to report that my seizures stop if I practice the following on a daily basis: acupuncture pen mentioned above, mindfulness, deep breathing exercises, meditation, limiting multitasking activities, and Vistaril (Hydroxyzine) every four to six hours or only as needed. My goal for the long-term is to stop taking this medication and rely on my coping skills.

I receive weekly one of the following: needle acupuncture, chiropractic care with massage, cupping, and dry needling at a local medical spa. I know this sounds overwhelming but it has significantly increased the quality of my life. It makes the difference between suffering and thriving.

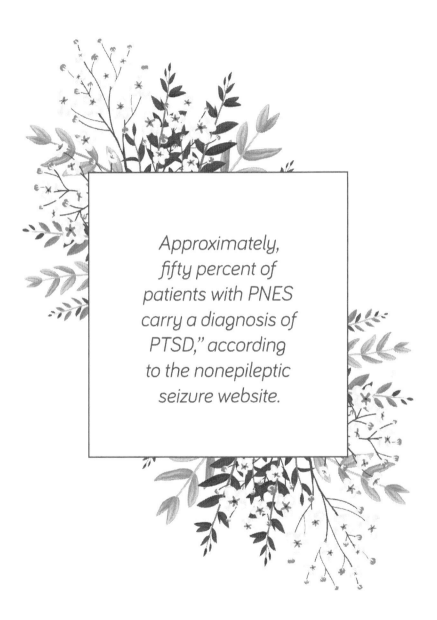

Approximately,
fifty percent of
patients with PNES
carry a diagnosis of
PTSD," according
to the nonepileptic
seizure website.

Some suggestions on the reduction of PNES seizures such as: "Distraction, counting backwards from 100, focusing on a conversation, singing your favorite song, reading a magazine, deep breathing, focusing on objects in the room, mindfulness, meditation, and reminding yourself that you are safe, according to the nonepileptic seizure website."[21]

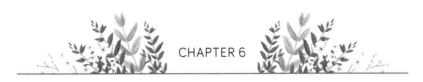

CHAPTER 6

STRESS AND ANXIETY

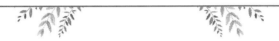

*W*e all know that stress and anxiety are bad for us but do we really know how much? I think my story will illustrate the impact of stress on our body and mind. For instance, stress can restrict breathing because we tend to hold our breath when we are tense. Over time, this can cause a decrease in our range of breathing, as well as damage to connective tissue in the chest/lung area.

Stress can manifest itself in many forms such as: forgetfulness, seizures, shaky hands, dropping things, headaches, brain fog, sweating, trouble sleeping, upset stomach, high blood pressure, poor sleep, and zoning out.

Meanwhile, stress can bring about thoughts of denial and frustration. I've even said, "I don't feel that stressed." After years of therapy, I realized that my state of anxiety was so intense that it was the only manner in which I had lived my life for the past thirty-five years. It was all I had ever known. I simply knew no other way.

My therapist told me that I lived in survival mode for so many years that I ran on autopilot. After I became ill with GBS in 2014, it gave me time to slow down and actually live in the present. I had lived in a dissociative state for so long that I had trouble expressing my emotions and feelings. I was surviving but far from thriving.

There were huge chunks of time that I don't remember and other things remembered from age three. It's interesting what memories the brain keeps active and which ones are repressed. The flight or fight response was activated.

I often had dreams of my childhood, which revealed unprocessed and traumatic thoughts. We examined these dreams in my weekly talk therapy sessions with my therapist. She was able to interpret them for me.

Stress management plays a huge role in cognitive function. For example, on a good day where my stress was managed with meditation and exercise; I calculated math in my head. I tested this theory while arriving at the answer to my son's math problem in my head without a pen or paper. This was something that I wasn't capable of in school.

My level of "brain fog" had intensified over the years. The feeling that I had a word in my head but I can't get it out. Also, distractions couldn't successfully be managed, causing sensory overload. Sights and sounds were too much at times requiring ear plugs and tinted glasses. Sometimes on difficult days, I wear ear protection muffs made for shooting because the over the counter (OTC) earplugs weren't sufficient.

Other days, words were stuck in my head but weren't coming out of my mouth. There was a ten to thirty second delay before I voiced them. Sometimes I pointed at things and had my family guess what I was trying to say. My son laughed and called it "playing charades".

I felt guilty that my son had to put up with a mom like myself. This was more than the average "mom guilt" that most women have. The fear that we will royally mess up our kids. I was jealous of other moms that were able to run, jump, or play with their kids. Years later, I realized I can do those things with modifications, but first I had to believe I was capable.

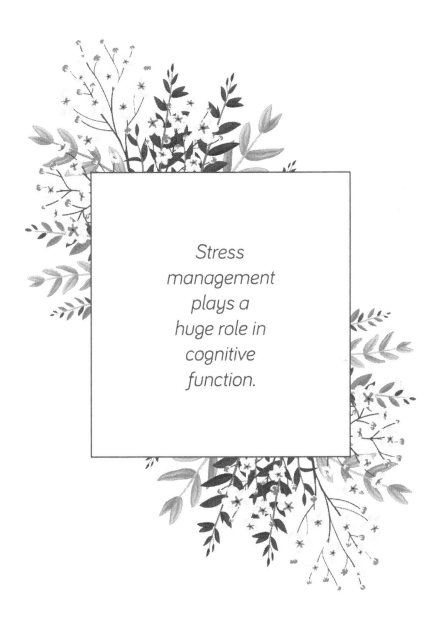

Stress management plays a huge role in cognitive function.

Later, I realized it had taught him valuable communication skills. It taught him to have a compassionate and generous spirit. Many adults have commented on how sweet, patient, and kind my son is. He even received a citizenship award at school for his kindness and willingness to help others.

Furthermore, my family's frustration grew when I asked them to repeat things over and over. I was so zoned out that I couldn't concentrate. This often occurred due to sensory overload from loud noises, bright lights, and interruptions. I had trouble transitioning between activities so structure was very important for me.

Routine is crucial to the management of sensory overload. I use a large whiteboard to plan my week. I actually check off items as I complete them. The key is to give yourself grace on the difficult days where not much can be accomplished. Remind yourself that you are doing the best you can at that time.

I followed a list of daily activities and routines that I tried to complete at the same time each day. This is helpful for when you walk into a room but can't remember why. For example, my mother used to search everywhere for her dish towel and I would find it in the freezer. She was so stressed she didn't know where she placed it. It's similar to driving somewhere but not remembering how you got there.

Finally, I have found the humor in it and learned to laugh at myself. It used to make me cry. I thought I had literally lost my mind. I was reminded of when my mom used to quote Mark Twain, "Of all the things I've lost, I miss my mind the most."

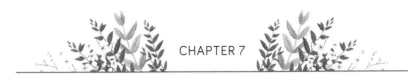

CHAPTER 7

FIBROMYALGIA

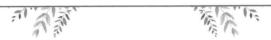

*A*s defined as a chronic disorder characterized by widespread musculoskeletal pain, fatigue, and tenderness. It's also called fibro. In most cases, it's lifelong or lasting for years. I was diagnosed eleven years ago.

Fibro is hell on earth. The pain is relentless. For many, it marks the beginning of chronic pain. This diagnosis is devastating and debilitating for many.

There is a long list of symptoms but most common are:

- widespread pain (joint, muscle, and nerve)

- temperature sensitivity

- severe fatigue/loss of energy

- sleep disturbance

- depression/anxiety (link to trauma)

- neuropathy

- intense brain fog (known as "fibro fog")

- tingling and numbness

- muscle twitching and spasms with stiffness

- Stomach upset (IBS is common)

- excessive sweating

- sensory overload

There is no definitive diagnostic test which makes it difficult to diagnose. In many cases the diagnosis is one of exclusion. Doctors rule out other possibilities by performing blood work and or imaging such as MRI or CT scan.

Typically, it falls under the rheumatology field. Doctors base their diagnosis on a group of symptoms. They perform a tenderness test where pressure is applied to 18 points on the body. At least eleven spots test positive for tenderness. Doctors use the tenderness test and above symptoms that continue for at least three months to confirm the diagnosis.

There can be extremely painful periods known as "flares". They can come and go. They can last a few days up to months. When my flare pain is around a "9", I feel like I am going to die and want to die. During non-flare periods, the pain feels more like a constant ache where you feel sore and sensitive all over. Sometimes, it feels like spiders are crawling on me.

There is a stigma with fibro that the person is faking or seen as lazy. When I was first diagnosed in 2009, this happened to me. There wasn't much support or information on how to cope with this horrible disorder. The frustration of "adjusting to a new normal" was devastating for me and my family. We all wanted to know where the healthy, vibrant person went.

Many people that I know with fibro, myself included, can pinpoint the time period when the pain began. Oftentimes, it began after a trauma. For example, my friend experienced this at age 11 when her father died in a plane crash. Some 27 years later, she still experiences fibro pain. For me it started during a failed spinal block, and trying to care for a baby with a bad back, and an aging parent to take care of.

There are three medications often prescribed for fibro that I discuss in the pain prescription chapter. They are: Savella, Cymbalta, and Lyrica. I have tried all three but only still use Lyrica.

These medications only provide some relief. There is no such thing as 100% pain relief from fibro. Lyrica takes the edge off but I still experience a great deal of pain. I still have to use CBD cream on every joint in my body twice a day. My doctor confirmed that a topical is best for joint pain and supports my use of CBD.

The singer Lady Gaga has a Netflix special called "Gaga: Five Foot Two" which depicts her journey with fibro. She helps raise awareness on how difficult fibro is to manage. Also, there are many online communities on Instagram. Here are a few:

#fibromyalgiasociety

#fibromyalgia.support

#fibrostrong

#fibro_warriors

#fibrofighter1

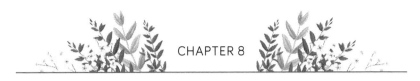

CHAPTER 8

TRIAL AND ERROR

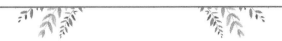

*A*s humans grieved by the human condition, we are in constant search for that "one" thing that will fix us. The truth is there is *not* just one thing. It's a combination of many things. "A trial and error process it is" as Yoda from Star Wars would state it. In my heart, I know the answers lie in the mind, body, and soul connection. Balance must exist between these areas in order to live in harmony.

This book approaches this connection with an integrated approach to healing the entire body and mind from the inside out. Humans spend a significant amount of time working on the outside of the body, often at the expense of our mind. We live in a put out "fires" society so that we only address issues when they reach crisis status.

Daily maintenance of the mind via meditation, yoga, and a gratitude process can keep things from reaching a crisis situation. We need to think of our mind like we do about our cars. Cars require constant attention and maintenance in order to perform at their peak performance.

Our mind works the same way. Sometimes the best solution is the easiest one. There is something inside us that talks us out of it with thoughts like "That is too easy to be the solution." Perhaps we over complicate the decision making process, I know I do.

Humans have the power to heal the mind and body. Unfortunately, this is a hard concept to accept. Especially, if we have suffered with a mental and or physical illness for years. This healing process requires a lot of work and a lot of patience. That's something that modern living is in short supply of.

This journey is not for the weak of heart. It requires turning off the noise of the world for a few moments throughout the day to practice mindfulness and meditation. For example, I tell my son, "Remember the importance of quiet time daily, whether you sleep or not, lay in a quiet, dark room for 20 minutes."

Furthermore, it requires soul searching and reassessing what we really believe and *why* we believe it. Due to unresolved emotional trauma, finding my "why" required years of "talk therapy" counseling once or twice a week. I even used some unconventional approaches such as eye movement desensitization (EMDR) and "tapping", which will be described in the next few chapters.

Moreover, I felt that traditional "talk therapy" with my licensed professional counselor (LPC) or licensed clinical social worker (LCSW) wasn't all I needed. I started researching alternative treatments. Next, I discuss my experience with these life changing treatments.

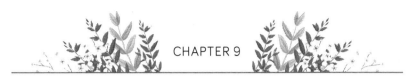

CHAPTER 9

EYE MOVEMENT DESENSITIZATION AND REPROCESSING (EMDR)

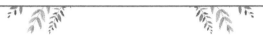

*E*MDR is a psychotherapy treatment that was originally designed to alleviate the distress associated with traumatic memories. It's especially helpful for working through post traumatic stress disorder (PTSD). This technique is often used with war veterans or individuals dealing with abuse. There are various methods used.

My experience involved a handheld device that sends electrical impulses to the fingers as it pulses back and forth from one hand to another. The patient simply holds the electrodes while the administrator or therapist adjusts the speed of the impulses. The therapist will ask questions about the unresolved trauma and ask about the details.

The experience is like a shovel digging in your brain. It digs "real" deep in the inner recesses of the mind in order to recall thoughts that were either repressed or have remained unprocessed. I felt mine were repressed for survival sake. However, at the same time these unresolved thoughts were slowly destroying me. It was time to face them.

The results were remarkable! After three sessions, I was surprised at the results. I was able to recall a repressed memory from childhood and reprocess it in a healthy manner in a safe space. Research suggests that even after one session, improvement can be seen. It's an inexpensive treatment that I hope will be used more frequently in the psychiatry profession. I have a friend that was assaulted and she had great results with EMDR in processing trauma.

Meanwhile, I think EMDR can be helpful for less traumatic events. It can be anything that has remained unresolved for years. For example, difficult relationships, death of parents, and divorce, etc. You don't have to be a combat veteran to experience PTSD.

Repression is a way that we filter unwanted feelings and memories from our mind. According to Marissa Brassfield at Realistic Recovery, explains that, "A person with a history of traumatic relationships may harbor pieces of this pain in their subconscious. Even if these realizations don't come to the forefront of his/her consciousness, he/she stores them internally. Similarly, a person that was abused as a child may not recall these unpleasant memories until forced to talk about it."[14]

Author, Brene Brown, talks about feeling numb in her 10 year research on connection, shame, disconnection, and vulnerability in her book "Daring Greatly". She discusses that unpleasant emotions can be numbed. However, when you numb, you numb everything. For example, we are the most in debt, obese, medicated, and addicted adults in U.S. history. She offers four solutions to living vulnerable and stop controlling and predicting.

1. Let ourselves be seen. Deeply seen. Vulnerably seen.

2. Love with our whole hearts, with no guarantee.

3. Practice gratitude and joy in the face of doubts and terror.

4. And remember: I AM ENOUGH

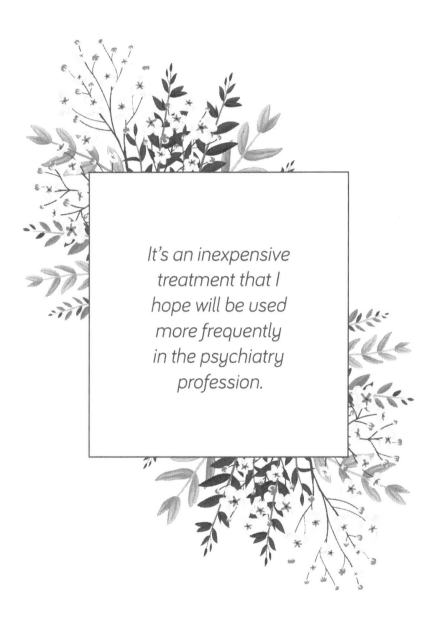

It's an inexpensive treatment that I hope will be used more frequently in the psychiatry profession.

My wish is for more people to discover the power of EMDR. It's such a simple technique to re-process trauma. In one of my sessions, I was able to remember the details of my attack such as what clothes the attacker was wearing and where the assault took place. I had repressed these memories for thirty-five years. My mind knew something bad had happened, when I was eight years old. However, I couldn't remember the details.

After listening to a friend's story of sexual assault, I gradually started to piece details together. Via EMDR, my mind was able to re-process the details and come to terms with them. The secret was to allow full processing, holding nothing back.

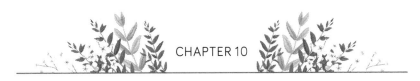

CHAPTER 10

TAPPING

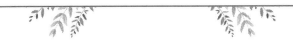

*T*apping is one of the easiest and affordable solutions to relieve stress and anxiety. And yet not many people know about it. Tapping on acupressure points in the body has been proven to reduce stress.

I highly recommend the book *"The Tapping Solution, A Revolutionary System for Stress Free Living"* by Nick Ortner. The emotional freedom technique (EFT) technique discussed in this book explains how tapping calms the nervous system. The balance of energy is restored and the brain is rewired to respond in healthy ways. Visit www.thetappingsolution.com for more information.

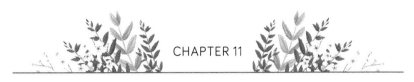

CHAPTER 11

BRAINSPOTTING (BSP)

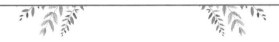

*B*SP is defined as a new type of therapy designed to help people access, process, and overcome trauma, negative emotions, and pain, including psychologically induced physical pain. The direction in which people look or gaze can affect the way they feel.

"According to the Good Therapy blog, "During BSP, therapists help patients position their eyes in ways that enable them to target sources of negative emotion. With the aid of a pointer, therapists slowly guide the eyes of patients across their field of vision to find appropriate "brainspots".

Brainspots are eye positions that activate a traumatic memory or painful emotion. It allows therapists to access emotions on a deeper level and target the physical effects of trauma." [5]

My therapist uses an old-fashioned pointer with a red tip (similar to the one my 3rd grade teacher used to demonstrate cursive). We have even had success using the pointer on video conference via the application, "Zoom". This is such an easy and affordable form of therapy.

It requires staring at the red pointer for a few minutes quietly. It helps me to focus and gather my thoughts. I sometimes do it with

75

candlelight while repeating mantras…combined with a hot, epsom salt bubble bath.

My brain resets. This is mind blowing. It seems too simple to be beneficial. Too good to be true.

We start our weekly talk therapy sessions with BSP, before we start talking. It helps to calm me and slow down the racing thoughts. I can do this technique alone as well by scanning my eyes left and right until I find a spot that allows my eyes to focus. I usually find a spot on the wall to focus on for a few minutes.

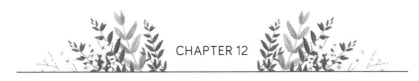

CHAPTER 12

MANTRAS

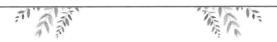

*M*antras are a free resource to help reduce anxiety, depression, and stress. Try repeating meaningful mantras to yourself several times a day. Set a timer to remind you. Many people combine mantras during their meditation time but it's not required. I like to recite them while staring at candles. The flame symbolizes the power of something so simple.

There are 35 mantra examples listed on HuffPost called "35 Affirmations That Will Change Your Life." [5] My personal favorites are "I am confident", "Set myself up for success", "I am active", or "I am bold." Another phrase I like is, "Expect and accept abundance to flow easily through me." A wise therapist once told me to repeat, "Let time pass" during panic attacks. I get teary eyed when I say, "I am enough." It has taken me 35 years to believe "I am enough."

Author Brendon Buchard, uses the word "release" as his mantra. He describes the process in his book, "High Performance Habits." He describes the process of inhaling the syllable "re" during the inhale and "lease" during the exhale. All breath work is done through the nose.

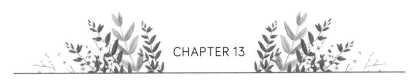

CHAPTER 13

CBT (COGNITIVE BEHAVIORAL THERAPY)

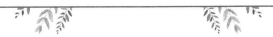

*C*ognitive Behavioral Therapy (CBT) is the gold standard in psychiatry. The recommendation usually comes when a patient still experiences depression even after being placed on an antidepressant, or for those individuals that need further psychological treatment options.

In my case, the nurse practitioner that was managing my psychotropic meds suggested I try CBT. We had spent months adding and decreasing medications. It was a scary process. For example, one of the meds caused a significant increase in my blood sugar so I was titrated off that. Another one caused suicidal thoughts.

CBT provides education on the role of the mind in the experience and treatment of pain. It explores the relationship between thought patterns, emotions, actions, and pain. Also, it addresses core underlying beliefs such as "I am not enough". This belief was at the root of my suffering.

These beliefs may be serving to keep an individual stuck in feeling hopeless or out of control with their pain. As such, negative beliefs can impact the functioning of an individual living with chronic pain. They can prevent them from engaging in active rehabilitation.

This was certainly the case in 2014 when I decided to give up. I slept 16 hours per day. I would numb out with television and binge watch shows for hours. GBS kicked my butt and I couldn't find a way out of my suffering.

For example, if someone believes that only a medical intervention will cure them, then they will put their effort into seeking medical interventions. The chance to regulate emotions via self-management techniques is reduced. I failed to see how self-help skills would benefit me. I felt permanently broken. There was no "fixing" me.

Chronic pain persons may also experience high levels of distress, when their medications are unavailable or treatment they believe will cure them is not authorized. Often, people become depressed or anxious when their surgeries or treatments fail. I was stuck in this mindset for thirty five years. I kept waiting on the next thing to fix me.

I was so upset that my back surgery had failed. My pain didn't go away. In fact, it made my situation worse.

Furthermore, I thought a pain flare up was indicative of my condition deteriorating, when in fact it was just a pain flare. These types of pain beliefs can trigger emotional distress, such as sadness, anxiety, fear, hopelessness, or anger. As such, it's important to address such pain beliefs to best ensure an effective response to medical treatment. Engagement in self-management principles is required.

CBT can assist persons with chronic pain. The thought patterns and behaviors that contribute to pain can be improved by demonstrating their self-efficacy for managing pain. CBT teaches positive self-talk to de-escalate painful cycles and trigger a relaxation response.

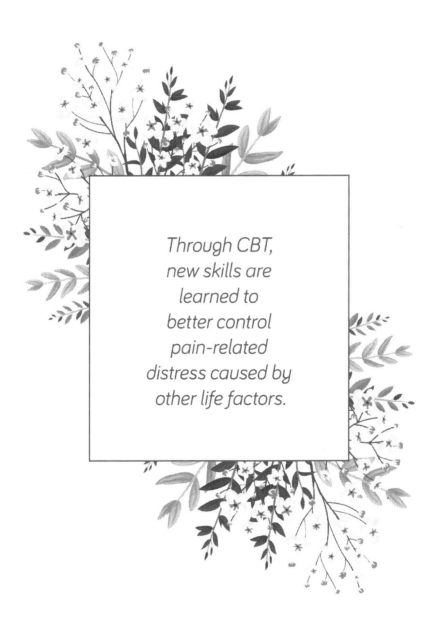

*Through CBT,
new skills are
learned to
better control
pain-related
distress caused by
other life factors.*

I liken it to the process of unlearning pain wiring. Chronic pain changes the structure and function of the brain. Years of chronic pain can increase pain sensitivity. By changing negative thoughts and behaviors, persons with pain can increase their awareness of pain and develop more effective coping mechanisms. It requires an integrated approach of moving, eating lower inflammation foods, and focusing on how our thoughts and emotions affect our pain level.

It's common for people to worry about their pain, which in turn causes distress and amplifies the processing of pain in the nervous system. What if we set time apart to worry and we only worry in that timeframe? This is similar to opening and closing a window on your computer. I have learned to only worry in the allotted time which increases the power of attention and focus.

For example, I have practiced this by sitting outside in my rocking chair with no radio or electronic devices. I rocked back and forth listening to the sounds of nature. I resisted the need to feel like I need to be entertained all the time.

Through CBT, new skills are learned to better control pain-related distress caused by other life factors. While CBT is an appropriate treatment for pain, it can also be used to treat the psychological factors that impact pain including depression, anxiety, and sleep disturbance. A combination of education, behavioral modification, and the changing of thinking patterns can help alleviate these psychological issues, resulting in improved functioning.

I have attended two different CBT programs in two different states, and found both to be helpful and similar in structure. It's nice to know you are not alone and that there are other people with the same issues.

The outpatient classes are about two months long and a manual is provided. Multiple counselors such as LPCs and LCSWs take turns speaking, as well as patients sharing their stories. There were about ten people in my class of all ages. It typically is completed in an outpatient clinical setting and is referred to as intensive outpatient program (IOP). There are also inpatient programs as well.

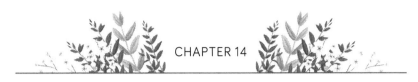

CHAPTER 14

DBT (DIALECTICAL BEHAVIOR THERAPY)

*D*ialectical behavior therapy, DBT, is a form of psychotherapy created by Dr. Marsha Linehan. It has proven useful in treating mood disorders, PTSD, anxiety, suicidal ideations, borderline personality disorder, eating disorders, self-harm, and substance abuse. She said, "Radical Acceptance means complete and total openness to the facts of reality, as they are, without throwing a tantrum.

She explains DBT as, Acceptance of life as it is, not as it is supposed to be."[7] She had borderline personality disorder and suffered from regular suicidal thoughts.

The goal is to address behavior patterns by teaching skills such as mindfulness, communication, regulating emotions, healthy coping mechanisms, focusing on one task at a time, and improving relationships with better communication skills and setting boundaries.

I found DBT to be more helpful than CBT because of the amount of skills taught. CBT is more theory based and DBT is more action based. I think DBT is helpful to take after CBT. It's a more advanced form of therapy. Participation takes place in a classroom group setting, individual therapy, and phone coaching. Role playing new ways of interacting with others and listening to others share their story is powerful.

DBT requires open-minded thinking that is flexible. Also, it requires letting go of "all or nothing" ways of seeing a situation. I'm guilty of black and white thinking.

There are four modules to DBT: mindfulness, distress tolerance, interpersonal effectiveness, and emotion regulation. All techniques focus on being "present" in the moment and not worrying about the past or future.

The elimination of multi-tasking has been the most effective tool in reducing my anxiety. By focusing on one task at a time, it allows me to be more present. Dr. Linehan refers to this as "one-mindfully." On many occasions, I have put my finger up to signal to my family that I need a minute to process my current thought, before having a conversation with them.

Here is an excerpt from my journaling exercise from my DBT class, "I feel empty and numb and very disconnected from reality. I had no idea what I was feeling other than pain. The pain consumed me. I want to create a life worth living but I feel stuck. I'm not sure how to show up for myself on a consistent basis. I'm struggling with my spiritual life. Should I give up on my religion or cling to God more? How do I find my identity again? How do I go from being an overachiever to barely achieving? I need to cling to my identity and not to actions. I need to feel worthy and enough without having to put action to the test."

I checked myself into an inpatient psychiatric facility for five days voluntarily. My psychiatrist recommended I take a DBT class. He also told me, "I think you have lost your confidence and if we can work on that, I think you will be successful. " At the time I went, I was in a wheelchair due to a fall where I had injured my ankle. I thought that the pain and poor balance was too much to deal with so I had resigned myself to being in a wheelchair.

He helped me accept that life had way more to offer than the wheelchair. I was scared to check myself into a mental hospital. I had seen the movies about what happens in those places. Are they going to put me in a white room and a straight jacket shackled to a bed? I had seen the movie, "Girl Interrupted" where Angelina Jolie was in a psychiatric facility.

My experience was actually a good one or at least not as scary as I had predicted. I did individual and group therapy as well as art therapy. There was also a minister who answered my questions about my crisis of faith.

I needed a reset button and a medication change. I felt my current antidepressants and anxiety meds weren't working. Life wasn't working. I knew I couldn't continue in this amount of physical and emotional pain. DBT gave me the coping skills to get my life back on track.

The days were spent coloring at a large table filled with women. We chatted as we colored. We had no access to our smart-phones, which was nice to get away from the world for five days. I pressed "pause" on my life and was able to successfully re-set my mind. It's one of the best decisions I've ever made.

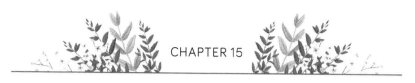

CHAPTER 15

DEEP BREATHING TECHNIQUES

*T*he reason I first sought out deep breathing was to help with my panic attacks. However, I was quickly amazed at it's healing benefits. The power of the breath is highly underestimated.

My days that began with deep breathing and meditation were way more productive and joyful. I began to watch instructional videos on the various types of breathing techniques.

There are many videos on YouTube. My favorite is *"measured count breathing."* All breath work is completed through the nose. This method provides some structure when a person is first learning deep breathing. I am naturally a shallow breather so this method is helpful.

Most of us don't know how to breathe properly from the abdomen. My PT, istructed me to walk while deep breathing and thus opening up the rib cage. This helped improve my gait so that I walked with less of a pronounced limp.

I use the four count method. Inhale for four, hold for four, and release for four then repeat the process a few times. You should feel an immediate sense of relief, energy, and calmness. However, this does take practice. It took me several months before I was able to do this. Now, I am working for holding for a count of five and working my way upward.

Rapid breathing also called "Pranayama" is practiced in Kundalini yoga. At first, I couldn't even do this for a few seconds without feeling winded. After just a month of practice, I can do it for thirty seconds without stopping. It's a great way to relax and to improve lung-related problems such as asthma. The pressure in all areas of the lungs also generates energy in all the nerve endings. The entire body is affected both by the breath and the pressure on the nerves. For more info on this technique and others such as alternate nostril breathing, visit this site:

https://www.kundaliniyoga.org/Pranayama

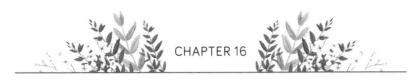

CHAPTER 16

POSITIVITY

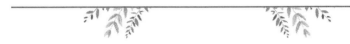

$\mathcal{M}$y next "life hack" is to listen and or watch positive content. I avoid negative or disturbing content. My psychiatrist said, "Stop watching disturbing content like "Criminal Minds" and "Law and Order". Those shows have a negative effect on your brain and mood. Instead feed your mind with happy and inspiring content."

I've never been a fan of "just be positive" as a motivation technique. I view it as a process not something you just "be". In my opinion, it's not an off and on switch. It requires cultivation and practice. I do believe there are some folks that stay in a positive state most of the time. I believe they practice "positivity" frequently or they have never suffered from depression. It places me in a negative headspace, thus making it hard to "just think positive."

The amount of television programs and movies with graphic violence is disturbing. Also, graphic video games with first person shooters have an effect on our brains. I think this is why we are seeing an increase in school shootings in the U.S.

This is also the reason I can't watch the news. I have a panic attack when I see the horrible things going on in the world. I dislike being ill-informed on world matters, but the sanity of my mind and mood is more important. My goal is to fill my mind with healthy and wholesome content.

For example, my joyful podcast recommendations are: author, Emily P. Freeman, called "The next right thing." She talks about finding yourself and tips for making difficult decisions. I also like a podcast called "Things Above" by Jim Smith.

The simplest solutions are often the hardest to realize. What if we have all the answers the whole time but never realize it? The solution is right under your nose. This has taken years to come to fruition. I think this is what people refer to as an *"awakening"* moment where the pace of life shifts dramatically. The light bulb comes on.

This new pace requires daily intentions. Being intentional on a consistent basis is something I deeply struggle with. If you struggle with intention, check out the Rachel Hollis podcast, Instagram, and books. I highly recommend her New York Times best selling book, "Girl, Wash Your Face."

Sometimes, I use my pain as an excuse to skip certain rituals like daily meditation or even taking a shower. Pacing is the single hardest task for me to manage. It's harder than the pain itself. The coordination of activities and deciding what is too much and what is too little to pack in my day is overwhelming.

Oftentimes, I would schedule an event or even just a coffee date way in advance then have to cancel last minute due to pain and social anxiety. This is where being intentional comes in. I make myself do things, even when I don't feel like it. Get up, dress up, and show up…it's that simple sometimes.

The difficult days require me to get ready in phases. For example, take a shower then sit and rest, then put on my makeup, then rest, etc. When I cook, I often have to sit down to chop vegetables, or break the meal into manageable steps that allow for rest in between.

Overexertion throughout the day causes a difficult next day with overwhelming fatigue. In addition, I now use a grocery delivery service, which I highly recommend. It will change your life! Grocery shopping used to wipe me out and require an immediate nap to cope with the fatigue. Also, I have a cleaning service that deep cleans my house once a month. I shifted my focus on things I can do rather than the things I can't do.

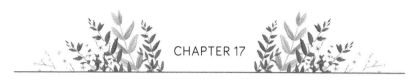

CHAPTER 17

GRATITUDE

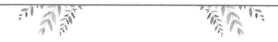

*P*racticing daily gratitude helps me be intentional. It keeps me focused on my life goals. Self improvement goals assist me on my path to enlightenment. Distraction is a useful tool to take my thoughts off of the pain. I recommend writing in a journal every day, at least three things you are grateful for.

Also, before bed I try to recall five of my favorite things from the day, that way as I fall asleep my brain is thinking happier thoughts. I use a small gratitude journal that is just for gratitude thoughts. I put it out where I can see it.

Life coach, Tony Robbins, says, "It's hard to be anxious or depressed when you are in a state of gratitude." I like his no nonsense attitude. He is intense but he is the real deal. He was homeless. He had a brain tumor. He knows what it's like to pick up the pieces of a broken life. His work inspires me as well as thousands of others.

The path of self development requires us to learn skills and tools to create the life we want. We also have to realize that healing is not linear. It is a roller coaster ride that never stops. We have to be grateful for all of the lessons or seasons, even the ones at the bottom of the ride. The magic happens when we turn tragedy into victory.

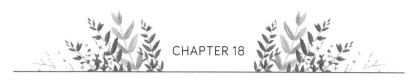

CHAPTER 18

VOLUNTEERING

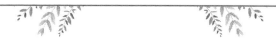

*V*olunteerism puts life in perspective. Giving back to someone is a good reminder of how good we really have it and also provides a distraction from pain obsessing thoughts. Tony Robbins says, "The secret to living is giving." To find a volunteering opportunity in your local area go to:

> www.volunteermatch.org

In a perfect world, all Americans should visit a third world country or visit the homeless under the interstate bridge. Volunteering at a soup kitchen or delivering food for "Meals on Wheels" will give us an enormous amount of perspective. The Department of Human Services and Child Protective Services are in great need of foster homes and mentors in the U.S.

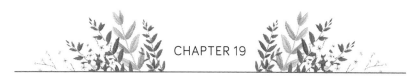

CHAPTER 19

MEDITATION

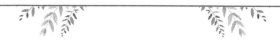

*D*aily meditation is a game changer. Life can only be found in the present moment, not in the future. My one wish for humanity is for everyone to practice daily meditation. Yet, so many folks refuse to try it. I've even gone as far as to meditate twice a day and I'm pleasantly surprised with the results.

The diagnosis of PNES came two years after acquiring GBS. My body converted mental anguish into physical symptoms such as seizures, twitching, muscle spasms, and sensory overload. That is why it sometimes is referred to as conversion disorder.

Meditation assists in keeping the seizures at bay. The days I forget to meditate, the seizures come back which proves how powerful meditation can be. Meditation is a life line.

Meditation doesn't require a fancy cushion, sitting in a cross legged position, or climbing a mountain in Tibet in order to be effective. I find it more comfortable to lie down in a quiet, dark room. I have found music such as "om" chanting to be relaxing. If racing thoughts are a problem, then a guided meditation might be helpful.

The music, binaural beats, use different frequencies to change our energy level and assist in the relaxation process. Twenty minute sessions are helpful when first starting meditation. The longer the better but time constraints might not allow for that. Several mini sessions per day are also helpful.

My favorite songs are found on YouTube. The first one is "om" chanting by Dr. Nipun Aggarwal.

The next song I recommend is binaural beats called "Happiness Frequency."

Meditation helps to turn off negative thoughts. Our thoughts and expectations can send signals to the spinal cord stimulating cells that either inhibit or facilitate the sensation of pain. The expectation of pain allows input from the tissues to increase the intensity of the pain we feel. In contrast, when we expect pain relief, our brain turns on pain inhibitory signals. Finally, our state of mind is a powerful predictor for how much pain we will feel and how well treatments work.

A Harvard neuroscientist, Dr. Sara Lazar, discusses that, "Meditation activates the prefrontal cortex, which in turn deactivates the thalamus, the part of the brain that acts as a gateway to pain. The thalamus can also regulate temperature, touch, and itch. The thalamus encodes information about the type, pattern, intensity, and localization of pain. She found a direct correlation between the thickness of the prefrontal cortex and the amount of meditative practice. In other words, the more experienced the meditator, the thicker his/her prefrontal cortex." [8]

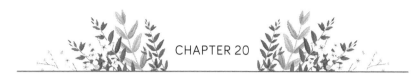

CHAPTER 20

BEDDING

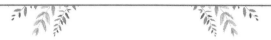

*P*illows are so important. Invest in some high quality pillows and blankets and even a comfortable mattress. The budget conscious may like the option of toppers and pads that can be added for additional comfort and affordability. A Tempur-Pedic adjustable bed has been on my wish list for years but I can't talk my husband into purchasing it.

Experiment with new sleeping positions. For example, I sleep with a large body pillow when sleeping on my side. This helps me from slouching and improves my overall posture during sleep. This contributes to less back pain.

I also purchased a wedge that elevates my head, neck, and back about three inches. This helps reduce neck, shoulder, back pain, and acid reflux. These wedges can also be placed under your knees, which helps support the lower back and can reduce leg and foot swelling. Wedges are also helpful for hip alignment.

My physical therapist said, "Get used to carrying pillows and yoga blocks everywhere you go." Therefore, I always have pillows, blocks, and blankets in my car. There are times that I have to lay down in the back seat of my van and rest or take a nap between activities. The long periods of sitting require a pillow behind my back and a block under my foot to help with my posture and pain reduction.

Weighted blankets are helpful for anxiety reduction. They feel like you are being hugged by sunshine. They are breathable and don't cause sweating. They have various weights. I prefer around a 15 pound blanket. They are pricey but worth it.

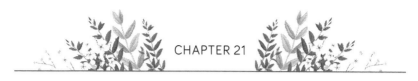

CHAPTER 21

FOOTWEAR

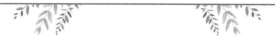

*I*nvestment of high quality shoes made for walking/running is important. Skechers, New Balance, or Brooks brands provide adequate support. Skechers come in slip on or tie in many different colors and styles so you can wear a "tennis shoe" with a dressy outfit. Check out www.skechers.com or visit a local "Ross" store or purchase on Amazon. These brands help reduce swelling and ache from neuropathy. Brooks shoes are helpful if you tend to walk on the outside or inside of your foot, they work to correct your foot stride.

Socks are way more important than most folks realize. I used to buy the cheap socks that come in a big pack sold at a local big box store. These socks get stretched out so easily and start bunching in your shoe causing calluses and or blisters. Invest in high quality socks like runners socks. Skechers make a great thin sock that holds up well after washing and all day wear.

I noticed that if I keep socks on all day and keep my feet at a constant temperature, then the neuropathy pain is less intense. Sherpa socks are beneficial for temperature control without sweating. They are available at Walgreen's or on Amazon.

Compression socks reduce swelling, increase circulation, and ease neuropathy pain. Amazon sells a brand, "Sockwell", that has many levels of compression. I recommend a graduated compression of 15-20mmHg, which is considered a moderate compression. They sell for $13.99-$24.99/per pair. These are especially helpful if you stand or walk a lot during the day. Doctors recommend them for flying to reduce swelling.

Flip flops should be avoided if you have neuropathy and have trouble feeling your feet. I can't feel my feet so I often trip and don't realize it until I look down and see a broken toenail and or blood.

Also, swim shoes are nice for water outings. There are many flip flops with arch support and thicker soles. Nike and Underarmour make nice slip on flip flops called "slides". Slides are comfortable because they don't squeeze against the foot. The "squeezing" can cause increased sensitivity for fibromyalgia and neuropathy folks.

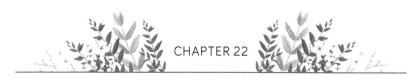

CHAPTER 22

NEUROPATHY

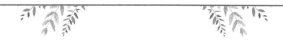

*T*here aren't many things that help with neuropathy especially if your case is severe. My doctors prescribe Lyrica (Pregablin) for nerve pain associated with neuropathy. I had tried Gabapentin (Neurotin) first but it didn't work for me but has shown to be effective for many patients. Typically, opioids aren't effective for managing neuropathic pain. See the medication section below for non-opioid medications used to treat neuropathy.

Ice and heat packs are helpful. I had a podiatrist prescribe some medicated cream with Lidocaine. The cream was not effective for me. She also mentioned rubbing your legs/feet with the lotion at least three times a day which was hard for me because my skin was so sensitive at times that I couldn't stand to touch my feet. Cannabis (CBD) products help more than over the counter products like "Biofreeze".

Weather changes and stress can bring upon different intensities of pain with neuropathy. During hot summer temperatures, my feet hurt less compared to the winter months. Humidity causes swelling as blood vessels expand causing increased pain for me. Barometric pressure changes like before a storm comes in can increase pain.

Neuropathy pain is worse at night because it can flare at rest. Neuropathic pain can come on at any time or in spurts. Mine is worse after exercise. It can range in intensity from mild to severe and disabling. Shooting pains take my breath away.

The burning and tingling pain of the limbs is referred to as peripheral neuropathy. Small fiber neuropathy is a type of peripheral neuropathy. The most common cause of this stems from diabetes and fibromyalgia. Peripheral neuropathies affect the peripheral nervous system. This includes the nerves outside of the brain and spinal cord. With small fiber neuropathy, the narrow nerve fibers of the peripheral nervous system are affected.

The diagnostic test to confirm small fiber neuropathy is a skin biopsy. I had to ask my doctor about it. I was surprised that I had to ask for the test and wondered why the many doctors I had seen had not mentioned it. Many of my doctors never explained the difference between small and large fiber neuropathy let alone what each one means.

Unfortunately, many doctors prescribe prescriptions like Lyrica and Gabapentin without performing this diagnostic test. The patients complain of the burning and tingling pain in their hands and feet and are usually prescribed Gabapentin as a first line of defense.

The *Skin Biopsy For Small Fiber Neuropathy* article by the Cleveland Clinic states, "Small fibers travel too slow and their conduction responses can't be captured by a nerve conduction study, electromyography (EMG test). EMG is a routine test performed to evaluate for large sensory and motor nerve fibers. A skin biopsy test is minimally invasive and doesn't hurt much and only takes about ten minutes. Lidocaine is used to numb the skin. The biopsy is done on one side at three different sites; above the ankle, above the knee, and below the hip. It takes about a week to receive test results."[9]

I had several EMG tests over the years. They were very painful. The doctor placed large needles into my limbs and observed the nerves on a computer. The needle was placed in various areas of the limbs. There was also a tool that simulates a shock to the nerves. That one felt like I was being tasered or at least that was what I compared it to.

The difference between small and large fiber neuropathy is that large fibers manifest with loss of joint position and sensory information, which can cause impaired balance and coordination. Small fiber manifests with the impairment of pain, temperature, and autonomic functions. For example, my small fiber test results are consistent with my symptoms of ice cold feet with burning sensations. It also feels like I have a large stone stuck under my toes.

My test results showed significant small fiber neuropathy. This means I have trouble regulating my body temperature. I am either crazy freezing or crazy sweating. I'm never just at a comfortable temperature. I have hot flashes and cold spells.

Also, I can fill an entire bathtub with hot water and get in without it feeling too hot. My doctor also examined my feet and found a diminished pulse rate due to the neuropathy and the nerve damage done by Guillain-Barre (GBS), herniated disc, diabetes, and epidural performed at time of c-section.

Also, during my c-section, a nerve block was used and the anesthesiologist placed the needle in the wrong area. This caused permanent damage to my right foot. I remember walking out of the hospital with my newborn limping. Doctors also said I had diabetic neuropathy, which started with gestational diabetes.

Furthermore, pre-diabetes can also cause neuropathy as stated by many of the neurologists I have seen. This is why it's so important to manage blood sugars.

Therefore, all of these factors contribute to why I can no longer feel my feet and often trip or fall. I often get cuts, scrapes, and

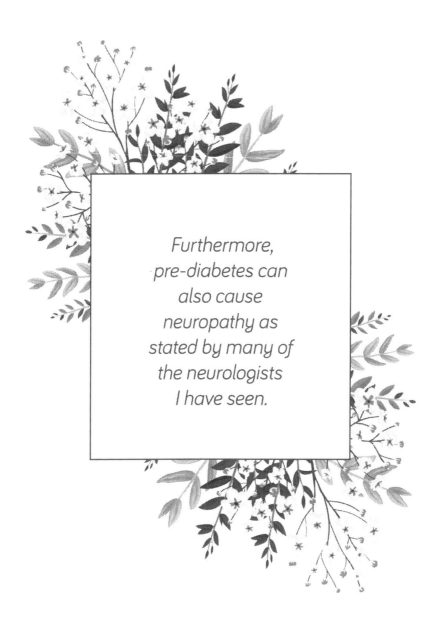

Furthermore, pre-diabetes can also cause neuropathy as stated by many of the neurologists I have seen.

bruises on my feet and don't realize until I see the discoloration. I have learned not to wear cheap flip-flops that bend. In the summer, I purchase high quality sandals with arch support. My favorite brand is "Earth Spirit".

Some easy ways to manage neuropathic pain are with compression socks. Also, Amazon sells socks with built in pockets for ice packs so they stay on easily. My acupuncturist also heats some heat packs and uses a velcro strap to adhere to my feet.

See my video about Lyrica and Gabapentin at:

https://www.youtube.com/watch?v=6Aw9x_zOkwA&t=115s

Neuropathic pain is difficult to manage but here are a few things that I recommend:

- CBD (cannabis) oil and cream (use one to two times/day)

- Massage

- Acupuncture

- Meditation

- Ice and heat packs (use for 15-20 minutes/session)

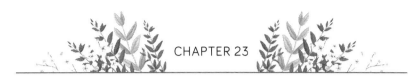

CHAPTER 23

MOVEMENT

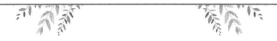

*E*xercise is crucial when dealing with chronic pain. The best advice I can give is "just start, just move." For me, I have trouble getting started with exercise but once I get going then I am ok, as I feel a spike in energy. Sometimes, I walk in my tasteful pajamas around the block because I don't have the strength to put on my workout clothes.

Exercise can reduce anxiety and depression. I noticed a huge difference in my mental state with 30 minutes of daily activity. I've heard many people use exercise as a form of medication instead of taking antidepressants. Five minutes at a time can increase endorphins. Sometimes, I break up exercise into five minute increments throughout the day.

A fitbit or exercise tracking app is helpful for meeting and maintaining goals. I have a goal of 8,000 steps per day. The fitbit sends reminders if you are idle too long and fireworks for completion. Also, I have measured that even on a bad day, I managed to complete 1,500. The more difficult days require a more modest goal of 4,000.

Getting started is half the battle. In my case it is more like 80% of the battle. The battle rages in my mind first. It's a catch 22 because exercise hurts but it hurts more if I don't. Yes, it will suck at first but power through and build a routine of consistent daily movement.

IT (iliotibial band) syndrome can occur from leading a sedentary life. It's extremely painful causing knots the size of grapefruits. It's caused my hips to be uneven which is quite painful. My chiropractor refers to the knots as nodules.

In my opinion, many doctors, physical therapists, yoga instructors, and personal trainers are unaware just how important IT band stretches are. There are many muscle roller sticks or foam rollers sold on Amazon that can assist with breaking up the fascia knots (also called fascia adhesions).

My favorite roller is the "Tiger Stick" that comes in several lengths. The large foam rollers are difficult for me because my upper body is too weak to remain in a "plank" position long enough to roll my IT bands.

The IT band is a thick band of fascia (tissue) that begins at the iliac crest in the pelvis, runs down the lateral or outside part of the thigh, and crosses the knee to attach into the top part of the tibia or shinbone. It forms from the tensor fascia lata and two of the gluteal muscles (gluteus medius and gluteus minimus) in the buttock and then stretches across the knee. The iliotibial (IT) band helps stabilize the outside part of the knee through its range of motion. It's the largest muscle group in the body.

I have found dry needling helpful in reducing the knots and less painful than expected. However, it does hurt but I feel it's worth the benefit. After just three needling sessions, my hips, quads, and knees felt much better. The knots are smaller and don't ache like they used to. Dry needling can be done at acupuncture, physical therapy or chiropractic offices.

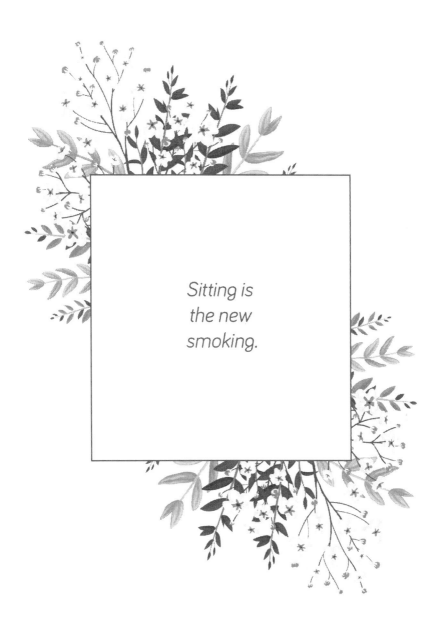

*Sitting is
the new
smoking.*

Furthermore, a sedentary lifestyle causes a host of problems. Sitting is the new smoking. The more we sit for extended periods without getting up, the more the pain increases. If you don't use it, you will lose it. I was amazed how fast muscle memory and strength decrease.

After one week in a hospital bed, I was so stiff and weak. The muscles start to atrophy, which predisposes a person to future pain. My doctor recommends stretching at least once an hour especially if you sit at a desk. Stand up desks and yoga balls used as chairs are new trends in the workplace.

Yoga, tai chi, and swimming are lower impact exercises that I recommend. My doctor recommends swimming in a heated pool compared to a cold one. Exercise reduces the sensation of pain by stimulating the release of the body's own pain relieving chemicals to enhance the ability to cope with pain.

Lifting low weight dumbbells and kettlebells twice a week increases muscle strength. However, it takes several weeks to get past the increased muscle pain resulting from working out. Find a way to power through and push through the pain. Ice and heat packs will be your friend. It will suck but it will be worth it. Physical therapists recommend alternating between cold and hot packs. Many athletes use ice baths but I am not there yet.

Furthermore, many exercises can be done from the bed, which is important after being confined to a bed for weeks or months on end. Also, I have done tai chi workouts from a chair. Focus on move-ment rather than fancy gym memberships, cute workout clothes, or elaborate workouts.

Focus on what you can do and not on what you can't do. Slow and steady wins the race. Small incremental change is realistic. The mascot for GBS (getting better slowly) patients is the turtle because of how slow the progress is. The journey is like a roller coaster with many ups and downs.

Finally, it's very frustrating when progress is stalled by injury. A popular quote reads, "Sometimes it's three steps forward and two steps back, but you're still one step ahead of where you used to be." Mike Breaux

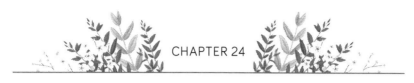

CHAPTER 24

YOGA

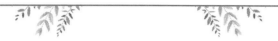

*Y*oga is also a game changer. It emphasizes mindfulness, breath awareness, stability, stress relief, pain reduction, posture, and flexibility. I practice three times per week. During difficult pain flare ups, I perform yoga in a heated pool.

I require some modifications based on my condition so I confirmed these with my doctor. She approved certain poses and would modify others. I have to avoid twisting exercises as they cause intense back pain for me.

I was 41 when I attended my first yoga class. I used to be terrified of yoga and believed it was something I wouldn't be able to master. I was never very coordinated. My mother used to call me "Gracey", for my lack of grace.

Start out with a slow flow method like restorative yoga or vinyasa. You don't have to be a yoga expert or very flexible when you first start. I was so self-conscious in my first yoga class. Then, another person fell during my class and I realized I wasn't alone.

Yoga blocks are helpful when doing floor exercises such as absorbing shock as one rises from the floor. Laying flat on your black with a block positioned behind your head can also reduce neck pain.

Turning your head from left to right can help stretch the neck and shoulder muscles. See my video about this:

https://www.youtube.com/watch?v=9UmyQp6lq_4

Personal trainers can be helpful for motivation and accountability. They can also verify your form is correct to prevent injury. I recommend the following trainer that is available for online sessions. I recommend Pree Poonati. He is certified in personal training, nutrition, and yoga. He can customize a program that meets your needs. He can be reached at About@nirvanagym.com or locally in Austin, Texas.

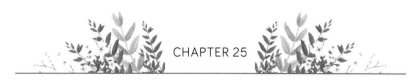

CHAPTER 25

PHYSICAL THERAPY (PHYSIOTHERAPY)

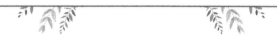

*A*l physical therapists (PT) are not created equal. Orthopedic physical therapy looks at the whole body. They provide customized exercises as well as proper posture training for walking, lifting, driving, sleeping, and sitting. These posture techniques greatly reduce the frequency of falls and can reduce pain.

My PT saw me walk and said, "We need to start over and teach your brain the correct way to move; otherwise, you will keep having the same issues over and over that lead to injury. We need to work on proprioception.

Proprioceptors are sensors that provide information about joint angle, muscle length, and muscle tension. Every injury has the potential to decrease your proprioception and balance. Balance can be improved with certain balance exercises. The nerves that generate proprioceptors are embedded in the tissues of the musculoskeletal system of muscles, tendons, cartilage, ligaments, and joints.

I didn't realize how important proprioception is and the importance of determining if my muscles will fire and complete a motion or reflex. My glute muscles weren't firing so my legs and hips took on the extra workload and caused severe pain in my glutes and hamstrings. My PT flicked her finger on my glute muscles to get them to fire. I was amazed that after a few seconds I could feel the difference. I felt the muscles "turn on".

A DPT (doctor of physical therapy) can be more effective than a PT with a bachelors or masters degree. He/she combines chiropractic adjustments, custom exercises, and "manual therapy" all in the same visit.

Rehabilitation doctors also provide this service. Search for a doctor that specializes in rehabilitation, posture, and movement corrections. It's important to find a rehabilitation office where the same therapist is assigned to your case each time treatment is needed. Rehab centers where a different therapist is assigned each time, is very frustrating for the therapist and patient especially in complicated cases.

Pain can be reduced by resting or pacing yourself. It's helpful to perform the prescribed exercises several times a day, compared to performing all at the same time. I remember when my therapist first mentioned doing the exercises four or five times per day. I thought to myself, there is no way because I'm struggling to find the energy and strength for just one set of exercises. It took about a year of weekly work with this PT to achieve four sets per day.

Water therapy in a heated pool is easier on the joints and muscles. The warmer the water, the better. Hot tubs (whirlpool) and dry saunas can ease muscle pain. Sometimes, I would perform some stretches in the hot tub because the heat soothed my achy muscles.

The sauna is good for releasing toxins and reducing inflammation. The sauna helped so much that I want to buy one for my home. The infrared heat lamp chapter below discusses how infrared devices can be used for healing. This is more practical when space is limited. Many spas and rehabilitation centers are offering infrared sauna services.

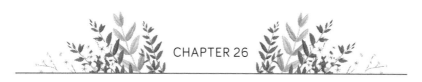

CHAPTER 26

SLEEP HYGIENE

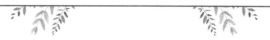

*P*ain can be reduced or maintained by staying on a healthy sleep schedule. Sleep deprivation makes pain worse. Keeping an irregular schedule without routine can cause poor quality sleep. Dr. Howard Fields, MD, PhD is a professor of neurology at the University of California, says that, "Partial sleep deprivation (staying awake from 11 p.m. to 3 a.m.) induced increases in pain, fatigue, depression, and anxiety."[10]

A consistent bedtime and wake-up time is so important. My sleep quality drastically improved, once I established a routine of waking around the same time daily and going to sleep at the same time.

My fitbit also tracks my sleep quality based on my heart rate and breathing. It categorizes the level of sleep (REM, light, deep, or awake) and how long was spent in each category. The results showed that I spent around 75% of my night in light sleep. No wonder I wake up feeling tired.

It's also important to limit the amount of screen time before bed or at least turn down the brightness on electronic devices. The goal is to limit distractions, such as notifications of email and text messaging. Experts recommend leaving your smart phone in another room.

Sleep can arrive faster by reading and or meditation before bed. About five years ago, I removed the television from my bedroom to reduce distractions and calm my mind. I've heard many doctors state that the bedroom should only be for sleeping and sex.

I've learned the hard way that repeated "snoozes" of the alarm doesn't make you feel more rested. In fact, it makes you feel anxious, drowsy, and less productive.

For thirty five years, I would snooze the alarm five to ten times before rising. I no longer snooze because I don't use an alarm anymore.

After I watched a video from life coach and talk show host, Mel Robbins, I decided to try the no "snoozing" method. Her YouTube video, "Why Hitting Snooze Ruins your Brain," she said, "Your brain relies on sleep cycles to feel refreshed and energized. Once you wake up and then go back to sleep, you hijack your brain and tell it that it needs at least one more hour of sleep. The key to productivity is simply getting up on time. Do this for a week and watch how your life improves and your to-do-list shrinks."[11]

Also, here are a few life hacks that can help shift your mind in preparation for sleep: drink chamomile tea, read for fifteen minutes, prepare for tomorrow, meditation, water on the nightstand, and reflect on the best part of your day. You don't have to pick all examples, just pick three and focus on making them a habit.

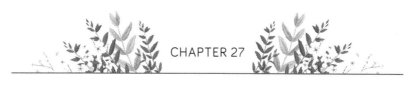

CHAPTER 27

CBD (CANNABIS) (HEMP)

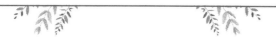

*The American Chronic Pain Association (ACPA) does not support the use of cannabis because it's not approved by the FDA (Federal Drug Administration).

*C*annabidiol oil derived from the marijuana plant referred to as CBD, may be one of the strongest, natural inflammation and joint pain fighters out there. It comes in many forms: oil, capsule, edibles, balms, lotions, vape using a cartridge, and sublingual.

Many vendors offer CBD without THC (tetrahydrocannabinol). THC is the "high" component which makes it illegal to sell in some U.S. states and some European countries.

CBD oil has trace amounts of THC in it (.3 percent is the standard amount allowed by law) in most U.S. states. According to the story on Vice by Elizabeth Brico, "We Looked Into Whether CBD Would Show Up in a Drug Test, "CBD is chemically distinct from THC, so it is unlikely that pure CBD would be detected in the average employer drug testing program."[12]

According to federal farm bill 2018, It changed federal policy regarding industrial hemp, including the removal of hemp from the Controlled Substances Act and the consideration of hemp as an agricultural product. The bill legalized hemp under certain restrictions and expanded the definition of industrial hemp from the last 2014 Farm Bill.

The bill also allows states and tribes to submit a plan and apply for primary regulatory authority over the production of hemp in their state or in their tribal territory. A state plan must include certain requirements, such as keeping track of land, testing methods, and disposal of plants or products that exceed the allowed THC concentration.

The DEA (Drug Enforcement Agency) and most local and state law enforcement agencies aren't really going after hemp-derived CBD, which is why you can find the oil in vape stores, in skin products, and in stores that don't require a medical marijuana license.

This is because most of these agencies don't have a crime lab with the appropriate testing capabilities, nor the budget to pay for the upgrades as of 2019. Therefore, many agencies are decriminalizing it.

In my experience, the THC component helps reduce anxiety and promotes better sleep. However, many countries don't allow the purchase of CBD with any amount of THC but note it can be ordered online so that would be hard for countries to monitor and regulate. It's also sold at local farmers markets and locally owned pharmacies.

CBD is a game changer. It can significantly reduce pain. It's especially useful for reducing muscular and joint pain. However, there is a limitation on significantly improving neuropathic pain. I have found that it gives me a fifty percent improvement with my neuropathy pain.

It's known to help cancer patients and reduce or prevent seizures. Recently, it's effects on anxiety, depression, and sleep have been studied and published. I've watched videos on parents getting a medical marijuana card for their child that suffered from numerous daily seizures, and in some cases eliminated the seizures. I've seen positive results in the reduction of my non-epileptic PNES seizures.

CBD purchasing can be confusing due to the lack of regulations regarding dosage. Check out https://honestmarijuana.com/ for a dosage calculator based on weight and severity of condition. [14]

My favorite online CBD brand is "Plus CBD Oil". On average, CBD oil costs around $39/ounce per U.S. dollars. It does come in different doses which can be confusing so research before buying.

I think the oil and cream are more effective than the soft gels, sprays, and balms. The oil is taken sublingually. Place oil under your tongue for ninety seconds. I take the oil once per day. I use CBD cream twice a day on my joints.

I have a local source of CBD cream that is amazing. It was created by a licensed massage therapist (LMT), who suffered from osteoarthritis. He is located at AcuStretch, LLC, in Austin, Texas. It's so amazing that I wish I had a machine that sprayed it on like a spray tan. He can be contacted at michael@moodangel.com.

CBD oil can be used in a vape pen and both can be purchased at a local vape shop or online. However, there were some deaths associated with the nicotine vaping cartridge. It's difficult to identify all the chemicals found in cartridges. Therefore, I no longer recommend the vape pen as of 2019.

Consequently, the great marijuana legalization debate continues. There is still great confusion about the difference between hemp and marijuana. Drug enforcement agencies and legislators are challenged with this dilemma. Pharmacy companies are still lobbying Congress to veto the legalization of marijuana. "Big pharma" doesn't want the legalization of marijuana because it would reduce the purchase of prescription medications.

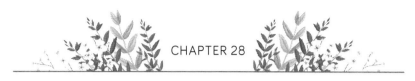

CHAPTER 28

NAPS

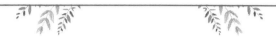

I experience nap shaming and judgement with comments like, "Must be nice, I wish I could take a nap." I have experienced that if I don't take a nap then I will fall asleep at six p.m. and miss out on family time. Fatigue is like dragging sand bags. I can't gain any momentum. Sometimes, I can shake off feeling tired by taking a quick walk, B12 quick dissolve tablet, or drinking ice tea.

I think the Spanish were onto something with their siestas. There are many benefits of napping. Naps can boost memory, lift mood, improve job performance, ease stress, and make you more alert. Napping or even just resting for an hour without falling asleep, can brighten your outlook.

If you are sleepy after lunch, you're not alone. The post-lunch struggle is real. A twenty minute power nap can help battle heavy eyelids. A nap as short as ten minutes can be beneficial, but keep it to thirty minutes or less because more can cause sluggishness. Compared to caffeine, napping can improve memory and learning.

It may seem illogical, taking a nap during the day can help adults improve sleep at night. Studies show a nap between 1 and 3 p.m. combined with moderate exercise like walking and stretching in the evening, helps improve nighttime sleep. I personally take a two hour nap and meditation daily between 1 and 3 p.m. Then, I go to sleep around 11 p.m. I have cured my insomnia by keeping this schedule and I can sleep through the night without waking up.

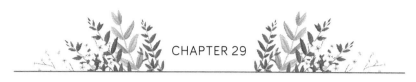

CHAPTER 29

NUTRITION

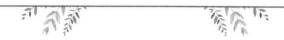

*E*ating healthy consistently is something I've failed at again and again. Nutrition is an area where I lack expertise, but I can definitely weigh in on what not to do. I have been overweight since I was eight. I even went as far as to have weight loss surgery a year after GBS. I lost sixty pounds. Unfortunately, I regained about fifty pounds within a three year time frame.

I'm trying to teach myself to take the time to prepare healthy foods instead of grabbing the quickest and easiest food I can find. My go to foods are easy, prepackaged and processed convenience foods, which I know are terrible for me.

Moreover, I use the excuse of when I feel better, then I can eat healthy. I'm not going to suddenly feel better one day without putting in the work to arrive at a healthy state.

I discovered MCT (Medium-chain Triglycerides) oil curbs my appetite. I had success using it in my coffee or tea. Next, adding more protein in my diet helps me feel full longer. Also, bulletproof coffee made with butter also aids in weight loss.

Next, I've tried intermittent fasting. There are many schedules available online. I use the 10-6 rule. I can eat between 10 a.m. and

6 p.m. I don't eat after 6 p.m. and not before 10 a.m. I find this easier than keeping a food diary.

For years, I have read books and watched videos on the importance of nutrition but still fail miserably with meal planning and execution. My acupuncturist recommended I do a five day mimicking fast by a company called Prolon. She had tried it and said it had helped many of her autoimmune and diabetic patients. You get to eat food but only the food that comes in the kit. It consists of soups, kale crackers, olives, nuts and seed bars, and an energy drink.

I highly recommend a fast of some kind every now and again to reset and renew your system. Prolon is easy because everything you need for 5 days is in the box and the food tastes good. I wasn't as hungry as I had anticipated. I experienced weight loss, less pain, reduced swelling and inflammation, and increased energy. However, it was pricey around $225-250 U.S. dollars. I purchased this at a medical spa and as of 2020 it's not sold on Amazon.

I purchased the Prolon diet kit on a whim one day after an acupuncture appointment. I used a technique found in Mel Robbins's Ted Talk and Youtube video, "The Five Second Rule ". "It states that if you don't act on a decision within the first five seconds, then most likely you never will."

Humans will find a way to talk themselves out of something or think I will do it when I feel motivated. Let's be honest, we are never really going to feel motivated so it's best to just make a decision within the first five seconds before we give ourselves an excuse not to follow through."[22] She also has many inspirational videos about this where she talks about "Why Motivation is Garbage." [23]

The internet is full of information on inflammatory foods such as sugar, dairy, and gluten. I know a few folks with arthritis or MS, who have successfully managed their pain and inflammation by simply removing these foods from their diet. My five day fast was proof of this. I am now a believer, you are what you eat. Put junk in, you get junk out in the form of low energy and increased pain. Finally, my goal is to make eating whole and healthy a priority from now.

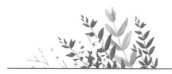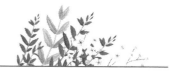

ALTERNATIVE TREATMENT SERVICES SECTION

INSURANCE

*T*he recent trend is for many insurance companies to offer coverage for chiropractic, massage, and acupuncture treatments. For example, my policy covers thirty chiropractic and massage appointments per year in 2019. The industry standard is ten.

Also, each chiropractic office and physical therapy center codes treatments differently. This greatly affected whether insurance covers the visit. It's important to review your bill to verify that the provider properly applies your insurance discount. I've found many billing errors in the past.

For example, many insurance companies cover massage if it was given at the same location as the physical therapist and or chiropractor. Many insurance policies cover a thirty minute massage on the same day as the chiropractic adjustment. However, they won't cover an hour-long massage session on the same day.

Also, my plan covered an eight minute session on the transcutaneous electrical nerve stimulation (TENS) machine on the same day as a chiropractic adjustment. Many of the coverage rules don't make sense. Research is necessary to find the best coverage.

For example, an appointment scheduled for a therapeutic massage at a chain store like, "Massage Envy", wouldn't be covered under insurance unless a licensed physical therapist or chiropractor is present at the same time. This information was rarely given unless the patient asked the provider's billing department or called their insurance company.

Insurance companies often deny a claim the first time. However, the patient can ask for a supervisor to begin the approval process. Don't be afraid to resubmit your claim. Persistence pays off.

Many employers offer HSA (health savings account) via payroll deduction or by an actual credit card for medical purposes only. It allows for pretax dollars to be put aside for future health care expenses. For example, if you know you are going to have surgery or need an MRI or other expensive treatments or tests, you can set money aside for them.

I hope the covid19 pandemic of 2020 will impact the healthcare industry in a more efficient manner. For example, I hope telemedicine will become more prevalent. My doctor mentioned that insurance companies might not cover these appointments after the pandemic is over. Also, I hope that healthcare coverage is not dependent on employment. Discussions should address whether a single payer system would be more efficient whether that is run by the government or private industry. I think there will be some important discussions and decisions that can improve the quality of healthcare in the U.S.

ACUPUNCTURE

Acupuncture is helpful in reducing pain but usually requires it to be performed on a regular basis for maximum benefit. Otherwise, the effects may wear off after a week or so but it depends on the person. I receive a massage, acupuncture and chiropractic services on a weekly basis. Sometimes, I think maybe they aren't that important until I miss an appointment. The result is I can barely walk due to stiffness, muscle, and joint pain.

The needles are thin and are placed on meridian points around the body. I don't find it painful but it can depend on the experience of the acupuncturist and your pain tolerance. Although, she tells me I have a high pain tolerance.

I recommend an acupuncturist trained in traditional, Chinese medicine. I have tried many providers but found them to be the most knowledgeable. My experience was vastly different at each provider so shop around until you find the right provider for you.

Currently, at Jasmine Acupuncture in Austin, Texas, I experience pain relief within twenty minutes of treatment. Typically, pain relief should be experienced by the end of your session. I have had sessions with other providers where I didn't feel any benefits.

The session takes about twenty minutes once the needles are placed. Sometimes, they fall out after the accupressure point is relieved. I think it is most helpful when combined with other treatments like massage, infrared light, ultrasound machine, cupping, dry needling and bloodletting.

My acupuncturist does all of these modalities in one appointment of one-and-a-half to two hours. Be sure to ask the provider what services they offer and which would be most helpful for your medical condition. Many providers offer a discount if you purchase a package up front.

I also tried electroacupuncture.The needles have electric current going through them via a handheld device with electrodes placed on the scalp. The provider can adjust the strength. It does help reduce and or eliminate my PNES seizures.

Needleless acupuncture is mind-blowing because it is so simple. It helps with my fibromyalgia pain and can be used on any part of the body and or the meridian points.

It has a crystal battery that lasts three years so there is no need to add or change batteries. This device doesn't take away the pain but rather changes how the brain perceives pain. The stimulation overrides abnormal signaling and replaces it with a kind of white noise.

My neurologist approved the use of this pen. I'm excited that I can perform this treatment at home. This will save time and money. The brand I use, "Piezo pulse stimulator pen", isn't sold on Amazon but my local acupuncturist sells it for $99 U.S. dollars. However, there are numerous brands sold on Amazon but I haven't tried them.

ULTRASOUND

A mechanical machine uses sound waves to target soft tissue via a wand instrument. It sounds like a jackhammer vibrating. My muscle and joint pain was reduced significantly. Thus, my heavy muscles feel much lighter. I found it very helpful in reducing back pain.

There are several types of ultrasound machines. I also enjoy the machine that uses a heat wand. It is helpful on my feet to help ease neuropathy pain. These machines can be expensive to purchase for the provider. My acupuncturist charges $30-60 U.S. dollars for a 15 minute session. This really helps reduce back pain.

The closest thing I have at home is a hand held device with a vibrating ball which is more affordable, around $40 U.S. dollars. The longer the handle, the better for reaching the back. They come with a set of shapes like, claw, circle, etc. for versatility. The speed can also be adjusted so experiment with the settings until you find the combination that works best for you. I use the, "Renpho rechargeable handheld deep tissue massager", found on Amazon.

MASSAGE

Massage is also more effective when done on a regular basis. I recommend at least one visit per week. Most insurance plans cover ten sessions a year. Massage is effective at breaking up muscle knots (fascia adhesions). Fascia is a band of connective tissue beneath the skin that attaches, stabilizes, encloses, and separates muscles and other internal organs. Muscle knots can be quite painful. Tight fascia can throw off your spinal alignment, increase pain, and change your gait/stride.

My massage therapist makes weekly house calls. Hallelujah! She combines stretching, cupping, Graston scraping, and restorative massage. There are many types of massage so I will mention my favorite ones.

My muscles ache constantly so deep tissue hurts too much. My fibromyalgia causes intense soft tissue pain that is widespread. Swedish massage is light to medium pressure and helps with relaxation. Hot stone massage combines light pressure massage with hot stones placed all over the body. Sports massage is helpful for an acute injury so the focus will be reducing the pain in the injured area. Thai and Shiatsu are more intense and can be medium to heavy pressure applied and in some cases therapists use their feet and stand on the patient.

Aromatherapy can usually be combined with any of these massages. Some therapists charge extra for this. I find lavender oil to be very relaxing.

Lastly, myofascial release is deep tissue for trigger point areas of pain and inflammation. The therapist uses their thumbs to apply pressure and hold it for twenty to thirty seconds.

LACROSSE BALLS

Lacrosse balls are helpful for reducing muscle knots. I prefer these over foam rollers. They are more firm than tennis balls so they are capable of providing a deep tissue massage. This is a form of myofascial release.

Fascia that is too tight can pull the body out of alignment and increase pressure on muscles, joints, thus, causing pain. It helps decrease soreness after exercise. Stand with your back against a wall with the lacrosse ball between the wall and the muscle group you want to work. This is helpful for those hard to reach areas.

I use them on my feet to relieve high arch pain and reduce neuropathy pain. They are also useful for relieving plantar fasciitis pain. They are inexpensive and can be purchased at a sporting goods store, a physical therapy clinic, or on Amazon.

CUPPING THERAPY

Cupping is an ancient form of alternative medicine in which a therapist puts special cups made from silicone or glass on your skin for a few minutes to create suction. People try it for many purposes, including to help with pain, inflammation, lymphatic drainage to release toxins, blood flow, relaxation and well-being, and as a type of deep-tissue massage.

There is discomfort at initial placement, but pain relief is felt after a few seconds/minutes. Some styles use vacuum suction, where the administrator applies a sliding motion on the skin and heats up the area before placement. I prefer the twist cups that allow for a deeper suction and no lotion or sliding motion is used. This provides a deep tissue stimulation and does hurt more than the lotion/sliding based modalities.

They can be applied dry or with lotion using a special tool. It can cause some bruising or red circular marks on the skin that go away after a few days. It does hurt the first few seconds as the cup is tightened. However, the benefits are worth it.

For example, Olympic swimmer, Michael Phelps, was videotaped with red circles on his back during the Rio Olympics in 2016. The darker the circle, the more inflammation present in the tissue. These areas also bruise easier and remain for a week or so depending on the level of inflammation present.

I had a frozen shoulder that was extremely painful for four years. Thanks to cupping and bloodletting, the scar tissue was removed. This increased my range of motion.

Bloodletting (see next section) can be combined with cupping. Also, fire can be used with glass cups but is usually discouraged for safety concerns.

Amazon sells some affordable "four cup premium transparent silicone cupping sets for massage" for $20 U.S. dollars. I highly recommend these and my LMT uses my own set. From a hygiene perspective, I feel more comfortable with my own set.

BLOODLETTING

This treatment has been around for thousands of years and was practiced by the Greeks and Romans. Thankfully, there are more humane practices today than in those times. I googled this term and many disturbing pictures came up. Oddly enough, there isn't that much info on Google about modern day practices and it's benefits. It can be combined with cupping therapy.

The wikipedia definition is, "The practice of withdrawing blood from a patient to cure disease."[13] The concept is similar to that of plasmapheresis where blood plasma is removed from the body, separating it into plasma and cells, and transfusing the cells back into the bloodstream. Both can be used as a treatment for dealing with autoimmune diseases. Bloodletting is much easier and cost effective than plasmapheresis so I hope it is used more in the future. I think it is a game changer.

My friend had scar tissue removed from an injured ankle and suggested I should try that for my shoulder. I didn't realize that this can be accomplished via bloodletting. The acupuncturist uses a lancet to prick the skin about five times. Then, the glass or silicone cup is placed over the area and left on for about 5-20 minutes.

This hurt less than the acupuncture needles. She showed me the "junk" that came out of my shoulder. It looked like thick tomato paste and about two tablespoons of scar tissue was removed.

I immediately noticed my shoulder felt better and I had an increased range of motion.

The question I posed to my neurologist about bloodletting and the needless acupuncture pen, "Is this hocus pocus?" She replied, "There is so much about the brain that we don't know, so if this is working, then by all means keep trying. It would be interesting to know that if you stop the needles and just use the pen, would it still be beneficial?" The answer is yes.

My response to acupuncture with bloodletting was that the number of PNES seizures were reduced over a month's span since I started acupuncture. She was impressed and wanted to share this info with her patients. Three months of use showed the seizures cease, if I use the Piezo instrument at least three times a day combined with meditation. The seizures come back if I forget to use the tool.

CHIROPRACTIC CARE

The activator tool is a chiropractic tool used in combination with back adjustments. My chiropractor demonstrated the use so I could use it at home. This saves time and money to be able to adjust myself at home. It has really helped my back, foot, and hip pain.

It's a small hand held instrument that delivers a gentle impulse force to the spine with the goal of restoring motion to the targeted spinal vertebra or joint. This is an easy, gentle approach to traditional back cracking from chiropractic clinics. I have had some manual spinal manipulations that were so harsh that I felt like a pretzel twist.

My favorite brand is the Original CAT Chiropractic Adjusting Tool - affordable thrust adjustment device sold on Amazon for

$134 U.S. dollars. I compared this tool to the one my chiropractor uses on me and they felt the same and delivered the same quality of adjustment. However, the commercial grade one my chiropractor uses is more durable as he uses it all day long so it can hold up to wear and tear.

HIP BRACE/BELT

My physical therapist (PT) recommends a hip brace because my hips are always out of alignment, where one hip sits higher. I have dealt with this problem for twenty five years. I've spent a small fortune at the chiropractor's office. Many chiropractors have a drop table specifically to adjust the hips, which provides immediate relief. My hips have been so out of sync before, that one side was two inches higher than the other.

This is due to my sacroiliac joint (SI) locking up and causing the sacrum to be higher on one side, thus making the hip higher on that side. SI pain is felt in the lower back and buttocks. It's caused by damage or injury to the joint between the hip and spine.

SI pain can mimic other conditions, such as a herniated disk. An x-ray of my hip confirms this diagnosis. Also, my PT confirmed this as well after spending a year with me working on strengthening exercises for the pelvis, hip flexors, and SI joint. She gave me a list of exercises to perform daily. If I miss a day or two, I pay for it. The pain is so intense.

The brand (Saunders-Sacroiliac Joint Support) is sold on Amazon. I highly recommend this belt for those folks with hip joint problems and SI/sacrum issues. I even sleep with it on. Also, a pillow placed under the hips can be beneficial during side sleeping.

The sacrum, SI joint, and pelvis are extremely important for spinal alignment, especially for women.

GRASTON

Graston is a form of manual therapy used to increase mobilization of the soft-tissue. It is one of a number of manual therapy approaches that uses instruments with a specialized method of scraping the skin. It's considered deep tissue and can be performed with plastic or metal tools. It hurts and feels good at the same time.

It's offered at physical/physiotherapy clinics and or chiropractic offices and usually performed by a certified PT or massage therapist. A plastic set can be purchased on Amazon (scraping massage board) for around $20 U.S. dollars. My massage therapist uses these plastic tools. I prefer plastic over steel ones. The steel tools are expensive but provide a deeper tissue massage. However, the steel ones are more painful.

Graston is really painful the first time but the pain eases after a few sessions. My fascia adhesions (muscle knots) in the IT band (thigh/hip area) were so large and deep, I cried the first time I had Graston. My philosophy on this is no pain, no gain. It really hurts but these muscle knots need to be released so the whole body is in balance. The knots can cause injury above or below the inflamed area. Mine were so bad it caused me to limp. The knots can pull the body out of alignment usually requiring a chiropractic adjustment.

INFRARED HEAT LAMP

This is helpful for muscle and joint pain, swelling, energy boost, and improves blood circulation. Many spas and chiropractor or acupuncture offices offer these lamps which can be used in conjunction with acupuncture. I have even used an infrared sauna at a spa. I feel much better after 30 minutes. The toxins are removed from the body.

The regular dry sauna at the local gym helps as well. There are also zip-up versions sold on Amazon as well. I plan to purchase one but they do take up a lot of space.

Also, I purchased a small desktop infrared lamp (Choicemmed 300 watt IR lamp light therapy) on Amazon for $55 U.S. dollars. I love it. It helps reduce my pain and gives me an energy boost. I use it 30 minutes daily with eye protection because it's pointed towards my face and neck.

This is a game changer. My energy level is boosted as well as an immediate reduction of pain sensations. I have consistently used it daily for 90 days and felt a huge improvement. If you don't remember anything else from this book, remember this!

I have Seasonal Affective Disorder (SAD) in the winter time so this is a great way to get a vitamin D fix. Many folks don't know if their vitamin D levels are low unless blood work shows it. In my experience, autoimmune conditions respond well to additional vitamin D. Besides the infrared therapy, I take 15,000 i.u. Vitamin D capsules/per day.

Infrared heat promotes the rebuilding of injured tissue by increasing circulation throughout the body. Thus, it can provide relief for those experiencing chronic pain, mood disturbance, and other conditions. My hope is that insurance companies will start covering infrared heat therapy sessions in the future.

TENS MACHINES

The transcutaneous electrical nerve stimulator (TENS) machine stimulates the sensory nerve endings and can assist with muscle and or nerve pain relief. The units cost $35-$100 on Amazon. I would spend more on these because the cheaper ones aren't as effective. The replacement pads can be expensive and they lose their stickiness easily.

I prefer the heavy duty TENS machine at the local chiropractor, it's more powerful. Therefore, I recommend it for severe musculo-skeletal pain. However, I usually have to ask for it at the chiropractic office and verify that my insurance plan covers it. My plan covers an eight minute treatment accompanied by a back adjustment.

It works by interfering with the electric currents of pain signals, inhibiting them from reaching the brain and inducing a response. I recommend it for nerve pain at a low setting. However, higher settings can over stimulate the nerves and irritate them.

The speed dial adjusts easily; therefore, use *caution* when turning up the intensity. I accidently turned it on to the highest setting and almost fried my hair. I compare the feeling to that of mild electrocution as experienced when I stuck a knife in an electrical outlet as a kid.

DRY NEEDLING

Dry needling also uses thin needles but differs from acupuncture in a few ways. The needles are longer than regular acupuncture needles. Also, it's more painful than regular acupuncture because the needle goes deeper into the skin to penetrate the muscle.

My doctor told me he had a patient kick him when the needle went into the muscle. All I did was wince. I seemed to impress them with my pain tolerance ability. I felt better after three sessions and the benefits remained. Thus in this instance, the pain was worth the gain.

It can be performed by a licensed acupuncturist or a licensed physical therapist. Dry needling focuses on neuromuscular conditions, pain reduction, range of motion, muscle tension reduction, and normalization of nerve impulses transmitted to muscles.

This has really helped break up the large muscle knots (nodules). It reduced the amount of shooting nerve pain that I have on a daily basis. I used to have shooting pains so intense, it would take my breath away and made me scream. This is helpful in treating my fibromyalgia and the residuals leftover from GBS, which is a neuromuscular condition.

This technique improves the signaling function between nerves and muscles. I could feel my nerves firing and jumping during the procedure. I felt my nerves "wake up" and start to fire correctly.

My friend had a frozen shoulder so her physical therapist performed dry needling on her shoulder. After a few sessions, she felt a major improvement.

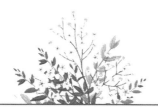

ALTERNATIVE
TREATMENTS

STEM CELL THERAPIES

*S*tem cells are the parent cells that can grow into any type of cell in the body. Stem cell therapies are becoming more common and available via clinical trials. Ask your doctor if their office is involved in one.

There has been a lot of controversy regarding stem cells because they were harvested from human embryos. However, the treatments discussed below focus on recycling the body's own cells. This is referred to as "transplantation" of cells where healthy cells are administered directly to the affected area. This can be accomplished by intravenous (IV), intramuscular, or by a spinal tap.

Stem cell procedures are intended to help your body heal injured tissue and are shown to be effective for pain relief. There is even a type of stem cell treatment called *"CAR-T cell"* in which a patient's own immune cells are harvested and re-engineered in the laboratory.

The Telegraph, U.K., talks about a successful stem cell surgery on famous golfer, Jack Nicklaus, "Where stem cells were harvested from his body fat (abdomen), and they were filtered and injected into his back using a local anesthetic. It was a quick 30 minute procedure and it cured his back pain."[14]

Furthermore, there are other methods of cell reproduction. For example, my acupuncturist recommends a five day fast to stimulate growth of new stem cells. A company called "Prolon" sells their fasting kits for around $250 U.S. dollars. This includes all the food needed for five days. The kit comes with soups, snacks, teas, and energy drinks and bars.

She said that it helped many of her diabetic patients reduce their blood sugars. It provides nutrients/vitamins that provide nourishment without feeling hungry and mimics the state of fasting. My experience with Prolon was good. I didn't feel as hungry as expected and the food tasted better than expected.

My pain level decreased about twenty-five percent and I had more energy than usual. It does come with an energy drink and a recommendation of none or limited caffeine. I allowed myself one black coffee per day on this fast.

The fast was the easy part. The introduction of regular food back into my diet caused some stomach upset for a week or so. However, I was eating non-plant based food so I'm sure the results would have been better if I had maintained a plant based diet afterwards or a diet free of sugar and gluten.

I still struggle with switching to plant based diets or low carb ones such as keto, or "Whole30 Program." This proved to me that an anti-inflammatory diet does help but doesn't 100% fix the problem. There is a strong link between what we put in our bodies and how our cells can regenerate and heal themselves.

My continued hope is to work through the reasons why I eat unhealthy and or binge eat. Then, I can clean up my diet and make it a lifestyle choice. The vicious circle of back and forth weight gain and loss needs to stop.

Furthermore, there is another non-surgical option that is similar to stem cell production, called prolotherapy. Prolotherapy is a procedure where a natural irritant (dextrose solution), is injected into the soft tissue of an injured joint. The irritant kick-starts the body's healing response. It's also known as a regenerative joint injection or non-surgical ligament and tendon reconstruction.

It's most commonly used in the following areas: back, knees, hips, and shoulders. In some cases, people with chronic conditions, such as degenerative disc disease or arthritis, can use prolotherapy to help ease their pain. Supporters believe that it may provide significant pain relief for joint or back pain. Costs seem to range from around $250 to $600 for the procedure. The exact cost depends on the site of the injections, who performs the treatment, and if any additional treatment is required." It's typically not covered by insurance.

My friend had the shoulder injection and reported pain reduction and increase in the range of motion. She reported that it took about six months to feel a big improvement and wasn't covered by insurance.

SPINAL CORD STIMULATOR

Spinal Cord Stimulation (SCS) as described by Medtronic, talks about their new SCS device that is revolutionizing chronic back pain treatment. It can be done with an easy outpatient procedure. "It's an effective alternative or adjunct treatment to other therapies that have failed to manage pain. An implantable spinal cord stimulator delivers small electrical signals through a lead implanted in the epidural space. Pain signals are inhibited before they reach the brain. Instead of pain, patients may feel pain relief." [15]

My friend had an SCS surgery and he reported about a 40% improvement of back pain. I have also read about many patients stating that it reduces pain but not 100% but it does provide enough relief to get patients off opioids.

CLINICAL TRIALS

The U.S. Food and Drug Administration (FDA) approves a clinical trial to begin. Scientists perform laboratory tests and studies to test a potential therapy's safety and efficacy. If these studies show favorable results, the FDA gives approval for the intervention to move to the next phase.

Participants may find out about new treatments before they are widely available, by being part of a clinical trial. Major medical breakthroughs could not happen without the generosity of clinical trial participants. For more info visit:

ClinicalTrials.gov.

Clinical trials are much easier to find and participate in compared to ten years ago. They are even advertised on television now. I've seen signs in my doctor's office asking for participants. I had a few doctors over the years ask me to participate. The requirement to quit some of my current medications wasn't an option for me.

Currently, my husband participates in a clinical trial for an FDA approved medication. We have had a great experience and insurance covered around ninety-eight percent of the cost. He is on an 18 month trial that requires monthly lab work to track the progress. Therefore, they are usually a big time commitment.

CORTISONE AND "SUPER GEL" INJECTIONS

Cortisone shots are injections that may help relieve pain and inflammation in a specific area of your body. They're most commonly injected into joints, such as your ankle, elbow, hip, knee, shoulder, spine and wrist. Cortisone shots can benefit even the small joints in your hands and feet.

They are easily available from primary and specialist doctors. The cost is usually covered by insurance. It's an affordable option. I have received several cortisone injections over the years and I must say they didn't work for me. I needed something stronger.

Harvard scientists have developed a "super gel" therapy that contains pain-relieving properties and the gel is injected into your joints to reduce pain. This gel could make cortisone shots obsolete. *Bottom Line's Big Book of Pain-Relieving Secrets* explains that, "The gel releases pain-killing drugs only when the body needs them. When joint pain is experienced, your joints send out special enzymes that cause inflammation and pain flare-ups."[16]

MIGRAINE CURES

Migraines are a recurring type of headache that can be quite disabling. They cause moderate to severe pain that is throbbing or pulsing. The pain is often on one side of the head. Other symptoms, such as nausea, vomiting, dizziness, and weakness can occur. Light and sound sensitivity are common and usually require isolation in a dark, quiet room.

The American Migraine Foundation sat down with Dr. Stewart Tepper, a professor of Neurology at the Geisel School of Medicine at Dartmouth and Director of the Dartmouth Headache Center at the Dartmouth-Hitchcock Medical Center, He said, "There is a new "antibody" cure that targets the source of migraines by targeting calcitonin gene related peptide substance (CGRP)."[16]

This is the protein responsible for causing migraine pain. Many patients have reported that their migraines were eliminated completely and others reported a significant reduction in the number of migraines. Designed to target CGRP, the protein known for causing migraine, these treatments are the biggest news in migraine treatment and prevention in decades.

One treatment option was released on the market in 2018 called "Aimovig". Three more are expected in the next year and a half, migraine patients are asking if these treatments apply to them.

Dentists are reporting a new migraine device called "NTI". It's a special device that fits over your front two teeth and is worn at night time. Dentists explain that some migraines are caused by clenching your teeth together (teeth grinding) during the night. "NTI" is FDA approved and can be obtained via your dentist.

CRYOTHERAPY

I tried this once. I repeat once. It was three minutes of hell. I stepped into a standing coffin like structure and was blasted with the coldest air I've ever felt. I almost ran down the hall naked. I didn't feel any pain relief so this isn't something I would recommend and it's expensive. However, the app "Groupon" offers discounts.

I think repeat visits, maybe at least three would be needed to make the decision to continue treatment. I couldn't get past the first visit. It's essentially the equivalent to an ice bath. I have heard the actor, Mark Wahlberg, talk about his frequent use of cryotherapy during periods of heavy training for movie roles.

I want to clarify that I believe ice treatment is very effective. However, I prefer to get my "cold" from an ice pack.

HYPERBARIC OXYGEN THERAPY

This therapy involves breathing pure oxygen in a pressurized tube or room. It helps stimulate the release of substances called growth factors and stem cells, which promote healing. I've not tried this form of therapy due to availability of facilities near me and the cost but I've got it on my list to try. Some providers are advertising discounts on Groupon. This treatment appeared on a case of Grey's Anatomy television program. Finally, I don't have any real life examples that I've witnessed.

FLOAT TANKS (SENSORY DEPRIVATION TANK)

Float tanks are dark and soundproof tanks filled with a foot or less of salt water. Float spas are starting to be popular. Floating relieves physical pain and reduces stress and anxiety. Fibromyalgia patients report benefits in pain relief and an increase in feelings of overall well-being.

I've not tried this therapy but my husband has and he reported that he felt these benefits. It's expensive but many companies are advertising discounts on Groupon. I also have this on my list to try.

SUPPLEMENTS AND VITAMINS

- **Water** (drink ½ of your body weight daily) Dehydration is more common than we realize.

- **B12** (liquids are absorbed faster. My favorite brand is called "B12 Blast" by Bricker labs, sold for around $13 U.S. dollars on Amazon. B12 shots can be helpful for some but didn't work for me. I also use 5,000 i.u. quick dissolve tablets twice daily.)

- **Vitamin D** (10,000 i.u./day or get real sunshine) Getting daily sunshine is a game changer! **Infrared heat lamps** help supplement in the winter time or overcast days.

- **Plexus pink drink** (for energy and weight loss)

- **Ice packs** (comfort gel pack sold on Amazon)

- **Heat packs** (infrared heating pad sold on Amazon by UTK)

- **CBD oil and cream** (cannabis or hemp oil)

- **Blue Rub** by DoTerra (expensive but worth it because it doesn't take much)

- **Turmeric oil** by DoTerra (turmeric is more effective if combined with a hot liquid and carrier oil such as olive or coconut oil and black pepper). I mix them together in my coffee. It can also be purchased in capsule form or as a powder (most affordable option) at the grocery store.

- **Epsom salt** (soak in hot bath)

- **Alpha Lipoic Acid** (antioxidant that helps repair nerve damage from neuropathy)
- **Magnesium** (helps with nerve pain and muscle cramps)
- **Potassium** (good for muscles)
- **Pineapple** (contains Bromelain which has healing properties)
- **D-ribose** (helps the body fight fatigue and muscle pain-especially helpful for fibromyalgia and can help reduce blood sugar).
- **Multi-vitamin** (contains important minerals and is most effective if taken with food)
- **Bulletproof coffee** (made from butter or MCT oil and helps keep hunger at bay)
- **Topricin Fibro Cream** (relieves nerve and muscle pain)
- **Cosamin DS** (joint supplement)

THINGS THAT MAY MAKE PAIN WORSE

- **Weather** changes such as increased humidity or barometric pressure changes increase pain. My pain doubles before it rains. My pain is worse before the storm, not during it. It makes muscles feel heavy and sluggish. I have considered moving to the desert to escape the humidity or maybe just fly south in the winter and spring.
- **Temperature sensitivity** with extremes like feeling very hot or very cold and can include cold extremities in the hands and feet. I never feel a comfortable temperature. Sometimes I have to wear two pairs of socks or gloves inside the house. A constant temperature is helpful. Dress in layers and use ice/heat packs to help regulate temperature.

- **Hormones** can cause increased pain especially during a woman's menstrual cycle.

- **Stress and anxiety** can increase pain levels. Stress can have a cumulative effect on the body.

- **Lack of movement** can cause stiff muscles so prolonged sitting should be avoided.

- **Poor posture** can make pain worse. There is a *"text neck epidemic"* going on now which is caused from staring down at smartphones all day. It's one of the leading causes of doctor visits. Also, poor neck posture can reduce lung capacity, thus making it harder to breathe. The average human head weighs about 12 pounds and the neck has to balance that.

- **Multi-tasking** can increase anxiety that can lead to increased pain. Focusing on one task at a time can improve mental clarity and memory and reduce stress and anxiety. In DBT training, it is referred to as "one mindfully."

- **Fluorescent lighting** can trigger migraines and seizures (use full spectrum lighting) and have light behind you instead of above, to prevent headaches, eye strain or migraines.

- **Not helpful comments** well meaning folks who say not so helpful things like, "Stay calm", "Take a chill pill", "Just relax", and "Just cheer up". For example, my husband sometimes says, "Wow you have the cat claw out today." Trust me these kinds of statements only make anxiety worse especially if the person is already dealing with chronic pain.

The reduction of these statements can improve the quality of any relationship. I also think it's great marriage advice! I'm not discounting the frustration felt by family and friends of the chronic pain individual.

There will be times when the caregiver is tired of having to deal with chronic pain and picking up the slack. Also, they grieve the more active person that is gone. The dynamic of the relationship has changed dramatically.

Let's face it, nobody likes to hear complaining especially when the individual is not engaged in active rehabilitation. My father was an example of this. He complained incessantly and refused to help himself.

I am not saying that complaining is never an option. It can be therapeutic at times to be able to vent or let off some steam. My therapist reminds me it's ok for me to have a "fit" as long as I don't stay in that place. My fit resembles eye rolling, screaming into a pillow, sighing, and complaining.

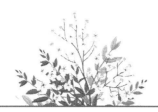

NON-RECOMMENDED TREATMENTS FOR PAIN MANAGEMENT

- **Cold laser** therapy wasn't beneficial for me. I had a chiropractor try it on my back on several occasions and I didn't see any improvement in my pain level.

- **Pain patches** are available via prescription and over the counter (OTC). I have tried both and didn't notice any improvement in my pain level. The exception is the prescription patch, Fentanyl (narcotic opiate), which is very strong and has led to overdoses. I had an allergic reaction to Fentanyl that slowed my heart rate and landed me in the hospital for two days. Therefore, use Fentanyl with extreme caution.

  Many over the counter (OTC) patches contain Lidocaine or Mentholatum. I have tried both. I couldn't tell the difference between the OTC ones and the prescription ones. Biofreeze and Icyhot are popular OTC pain relief gels.

- **Salt caves** are fun and relaxing. However, I didn't notice any change or improvement of pain.

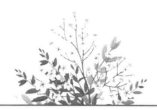

HELPFUL TOOLS

- **Weighted blankets** (reduce anxiety)
- **Distraction** (change of scenery-go to a different room or go outside)
- **Support groups** (remind yourself you're not alone)
- **Gratitude**
- **Grace** (give yourself grace for your noble effort)
- **Joy** (choose)
- **Pet therapy** (my pets help me get out of bed-they are my alarm clock)
- **Humor/laughter**
- **Half smile**
- **Body language** (do a power pose for 2 minutes such as hands on hips or open arms and palms facing up-see www.getlifemaps.com)
- **Radical acceptance**
- **Journaling**
- **Walk barefoot in the grass**
- **Find an uplifting podcast** (www.emilypfreeman.com)
- **Go old school** (board games, pet a puppy, or go to a concert)

- **Counseling**
- **Self-soothe kit** (put your favorite lotion or essential oil)
- **Devotionals** (positive content)
- **Pain symptom tracker** (see www. theACPA.org or choose a smartphone app)
- **Coloring books**
- **Arts/crafts**
- **Pillows**
- **Yoga blocks**
- **Note cards** (place positive quotes in your car, kitchen, bathroom, etc.)
- **Essential oils** (the brand DoTerra is my favorite)
- **Morning rituals**
- **Start a compliments file** (document the great things people say about you to read later)
- **Mixing up routine** (in small ways creates new neural pathways in the brain)
- **Pay attention** (to something you normally don't like brushing your teeth)
- **Go cloud watching**
- **Get out of your comfort zone** (introduce yourself to a stranger)
- **Unplug** for an hour (no phone, t.v., or internet)
- **Edit your social media** (get rid of negative people or things)
- **Inhale** (upbeat scent like peppermint, orange, or lavender)
- **Do a beauty scavenger hunt** (on your commute or walk)
- **Make a small connection** (with someone in service like a sales associate or barista)

- **Intention/goal setting**
- **Healthy diet** (avoid sugar, dairy, and gluten) these foods can cause inflammation. I know several people that put their MS (Multiple Sclerosis) in remission by eliminating these foods especially gluten. For GBS sufferers gluten isn't recommended.
- **Volunteering** (helping others can take our mind off pain)
- **CBT** (Cognitive Behavioral Therapy)
- **DBT** (Dialectical Behavior Therapy)
- **EMDR** (Eye Movement Desensitization and Reprocessing)
- **Make a list of fun activities** (you like and a list of mastery activities or skills)
- **Meditation**
- **Mindfulness**
- **Ice** (place ice in your hand to change your state)
- **Screaming** (scream into a pillow to relieve stress)
- **Bubbles** (blow bubbles to reduce stress or frustration and is great for kids and adults)
- **Sauna** (dry sauna can be helpful in reducing inflammation pain)
- **Take class** (photography, pottery, painting, etc.)

In addition, here are some helpful tools that have worked for me. I don't presume to think that if you try all these suggestions, it will suddenly make your life great and all your pain will go away. I just want to introduce the idea of possibility. There is an opportunity to find something that will break the pain cycle. However, the strongest tool is using the power of our own mind. What if we allowed ourselves to think outside of the box?

Some things work for some folks and not for others. My research is based on trial and error. Figure out what works for you and what doesn't. Come up with your own plan of action to reduce your pain level and boost your overall mood. Our brains work best when they are challenged to try new things.

This is an opportunity to rewire our brains and break unhealthy habits and establish new ones. Einstein said, the definition of insanity is, "Doing the same thing over and over again expecting different results." Remember to record your new routine with a diary of supplements, services, and or meds and any benefits or side effects. The date of trial should also be recorded.

There will be some days that the pain is just too bad to function normally. Listen to your body and rest that day. Get up and try again tomorrow. I know before my feet ever hit the ground in the morning, whether my day will involve pain. It's usually from the PNES seizures I have during my sleep. They cause me to wake up feeling very stiff and sore. Sometimes, it feels like I was beat up in my sleep.

Pacing is the hardest thing to manage with chronic pain. The balance between doing too much and doing too little, is a real struggle. I pushed too hard when I first went to the gym. Consequently, I injured myself and was afraid to try again. Two years passed before I was willing to try again.

Now, I am more realistic about what I can do and what I can't. For example, I can do two sets of eight repetitions with dumbbells while the rest of the class can do three sets of ten. Another example is that I need to sit to cut up vegetables for dinner. The key is to find some modifications that work for you. I break up my 8,000 steps/day into three big chunks and a few smaller time increments.

The point is to keep an open mind as you try different and new things. Also, it's important to give yourself permission to fail. Focus on the effort and not the outcome. For example, five years have passed since I started writing this book. My first few attempts failed but I stuck with it.

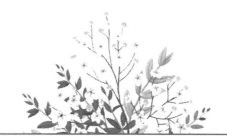

Pain Reduction Strategies and Resources

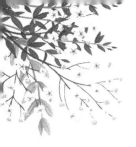

Pain Reduction

Lifelong complaints of suffering and pain,

But I choose not to live the rest of my life in vain.

If I wasted my precious time and the energy that I need,

I'd waste my positive efforts to succeed.

Legal, medical, and insurance exam horrors to tell,

But how is that to get me well?

Caring for my health is what I can do!

Relaxations, nutrition, exercise – forget complaining to you!

Teach me the skills so I can do my part

In order to have a better life at the very start.

Hard work, you say, will get me there.

Not life-threatening? That cost is fair.

So, you see, there's no need to complain,

Education and hard work will reduce my pain . . .

Beverly Sweeney

Moorestown, NJ

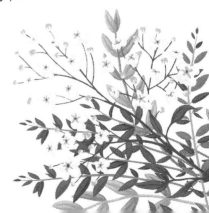

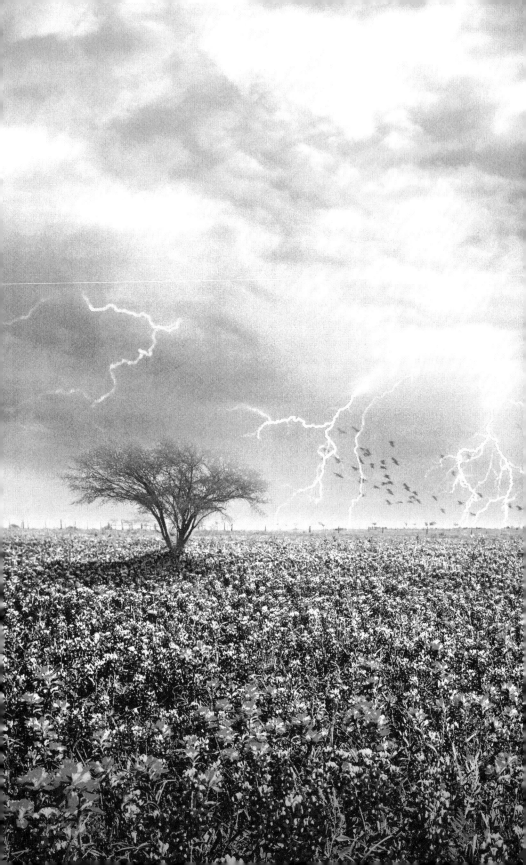

How to Have a Happy day
(by @thestreetquotes)

1. Slow down
2. Say thank you
3. Smile
4. Take a deep breath
5. Compliment someone
6. Appreciate small things
7. Focus on awesomeness
8. Notice three things you're grateful for
9. Stop multitasking, be present
10. Meditate

WESTERN MEDICINE

Historically, medications in the U.S. are over prescribed in our quick fix society. Medicine and healthcare services are big money. The holistic or all natural health care industry is growing. The grocery store chain, Whole Foods, has a strong market share in this industry. Also, many vitamins and supplements can be ordered online.

My biggest regret is that I didn't explore these holistic options before ever taking a prescription pill. Unfortunately, that was not the case. I had exhausted western medicine options before I was ready to try some holistic alternatives.

The previous chapters covered holistic alternatives. Next, I will briefly discuss some non-opiate medications that are heavily prescribed in the U.S. and that I've tried. I am afraid that if I use narcotics on a long term basis, I would become addicted. I have a family history of addiction. I stopped taking them in 2014.

The best option for me is a combination approach, also called integrated or functional medicine. It combines western medicine and holistic solutions. It's a trial and error process to figure out what works for my body.

For example, taking medication three times a day is more effective than just once a day. We are all different, so what might work for one person might not for the other.

I wish the side effects of these meds would have been explained by my doctor beforehand. I had so many doctors pushing pills on me with little or no information. My pharmacist was usually the person to explain the side effects.

The following medications are used to treat pain, migraines, seizures, depression, and anxiety and are often used congruently.

Many medications can have at least two names and or brands which can vary greatly by country. Therefore, use Google to look up all associated names.

Also, don't stop taking medication, cold turkey without consulting your doctor. Your doctor or pharmacist can provide you a titration schedule to slowly come off a medication. I learned the hard way on a few of these. My body required an even slower titration schedule given by my doctor.

Lyrica (Pregablin) is the only medication that I couldn't titrate or stop successfully. My feet burned with the most intense pain that I've ever known. Also, I had suicidal thoughts during the titration. I pray there is a day that I no longer have to take Lyrica. Unfortunately that is not today.

Also, I gained a significant amount of weight since taking Lyrica as well as thousands of other people according to online blogs and support groups. It's very frustrating that some doctors didn't believe their patients when we reported the weight gain.

I told my doctor about my twenty pound weight gain within the first month of taking Lyrica. He refused to believe that was possible. It has the same effect as steroids where you want to eat everything that is not glued down.

Ultram (Tramadol) is a narcotic that I have used only on a few occasions. It's a mild narcotic used to treat moderate to severe pain. The advantages are: inexpensive and effective at relieving pain. The disadvantages: irritability, drowsiness, and headaches. My husband called it "Damitol" because it made me really agitated.

I included medications most commonly prescribed for depression and anxiety, because it's been my experience that mental and physical symptoms go hand in hand. Also, these types of medications can be prescribed off label. This means they are prescribed for conditions that were not originally intended.

PAIN RELIEF PRESCRIPTIONS

Consult your doctor concerning these medications as each person reacts in a different manner. These statements are the opinion of the author.

NON-OPIATES

- **Hydroxyzine (Vistaril)** - An antihistamine that reduces pain, anxiety, and aids in sleep. Compared to Xanax, it's safer to take over the long-term compared to benzodiazepines. *Advantages*: is inexpensive and comes in a generic form and has few side effects. *Disadvantages:* dry mouth and mild drowsiness

- **Topiramate (Topamax)** - Nerve pain medication and anticonvulsant used for a variety of functions. *Advantages*: inexpensive and very effective at managing multi-symptom pain and can cause weight loss. *Disadvantages*: reduced appetite, brain fog (memory impairment and loss), fatigue, irritability, drowsiness, and dizziness

- **Savella (Milnacipran)** - used to treat fibromyalgia, nerve pain, depression, and restless legs. *Advantages:* inexpensive and effective at managing pain. *Disadvantages*: excessive sweating, headache, and dizziness

- **Lyrica (Pregabalin)** - used to treat moderate to severe nerve pain, muscle pain, and depression (a second tier medication usually prescribed after Gabapentin has been tried unsuccessfully by the patient). *Advantages*: effective for managing pain associated with neuropathy and fibromyalgia. It can be prescribed up to 3X/

day. *Disadvantages*: weight gain, expensive, drowsiness, dry mouth, brain fog, swelling, and possible suicidal thoughts.

- **Gabapentin (Neurotin or Horizant or Gralise)** - is a first line treatment for nerve pain, restless legs, anxiety, and seizures. *Advantages*: inexpensive. *Disadvantages*: weight gain, drowsiness, and dizziness

- **Cymbalta (Duloxetine)** - Prescribed for treatment of chronic musculoskeletal conditions like fibromyalgia, nerve pain, and osteoarthritis as well as anxiety and depression. *Advantages:* dual action, inexpensive. *Disadvantages*: withdrawal symptoms lasting weeks, suicidal thoughts, fatigue, and sweating.

- **Buspar (Buspirone)** is an anxiolytic used to treat anxiety and is considered safer in the long run compared to Xanax. I found it effective at managing anxiety in the short term but caused irritability as the dosage was increased and became less effective over time. *Advantages*: inexpensive. It's usually prescribed with selective serotonin reuptake (SSRI) inhibitors. *Disadvantages*: blurred vision, irritability, fatigue, headache, and sleep problems.

- **Xanax (Alprazolam)** is a benzodiazepine used to treat anxiety and panic disorders. *Advantages*: resolve anxiety quickly (usually within thirty minutes after taking). *Disadvantages*: high risk for addiction, expensive, can cause dementia if used over the long term, drowsiness, concentration and memory issues, and fatigue.

- **Toradol (Ketorolac)** is a nonsteroidal anti-inflammatory drug (NSAID). It works by blocking your body's production of certain natural substances that cause inflammation. This effect helps to decrease swelling, pain, or fever. It's used for the short-term treatment of moderate to severe pain in adults. It's usually used after medical procedures or after surgery or during a severe flare or fall. *Advantages*: fast acting by intravenous injection, effective at managing acute pain. *Disadvantages*: can't be used for the long term due to kidney distress. Also, causes an upset stomach and drowsiness.

OTHER HELPFUL TOOLS

PAIN DIARY TRACKING

This is helpful to track symptoms and print out and show to your doctor. There are many free smart-phone apps that can be used such as "Pain Scale". Use your own or use one provided by the ACPA on their website or in your app store. Here are some questions to track before going to your doctor appointment.

Symptom tracking examples are: describe the best/worst day in the last 30 days? Were you more active? What activities did you participate in? What makes pain worse? What makes pain better?

BEST/WORST DAY	TYPE OF ACTIVITY	ACTIVITY LEVEL	PAIN DECREASE	PAIN INCREASE

MEDICATION LIST

This is very important to bring with you to your doctors' appointment so you don't forget which medications that you have tried prior. Supplements/Vitamins are also helpful to list as they can interact with some medications. This is also important to carry in your wallet in case of emergency.

MED	CURRENT	PAST	REACTION

CONCLUSION

I hope this book inspires you to try some of the life hacks mentioned in order to make a custom wellness plan for yourself. Find out what works and doesn't work for you and document your journey. Learn to give yourself grace as you pursue your noble effort. Live from a place of gratitude. Fall in love with the process of discovering your true self.

Acquire the skill sets and personality traits to help manage disappointments and expectations. Remember to practice radical acceptance over and over again. Healing is a mindset that must be cultivated and nurtured. The process is like a seedling that grows when sunlight and water are added. The more attention you give it, the better the results.

The original title of this book was going to be "Grace, Gratitude, and Guillain-Barre." I changed the name because I wanted to expand it to cover chronic illness no matter the origin. Many conditions have overlapping symptoms and treatment plans. I encourage you to share this book with your family and friends, especially those you know that have some type of chronic pain.

If your city doesn't have a chronic pain support group, I encourage you to start one. Austin, Texas, didn't have a general chronic pain support group because most pain related groups were focused on a specific illness such as cancer, arthritis, etc. The ACPA can provide materials to help train you as a group facilitator.

Together we are better. My hope is we can all come together to create and maintain a tribe of support, collaboration, and kindness. Building strong communities can help facilitate the change that the world so desperately needs. You are that change.

You are not alone.

ALTERNATIVE THERAPIES TRACKING
(i.e. acupuncture, massage, CBT, DBT, EMDR)

TYPE OF THERAPY	BENEFITS	DATE	COST

AMERICAN CHRONIC PAIN ASSOCIATION

American Chronic Pain Association - www.theacpa.org.

They provide pain tracker applications, helpful videos, inspiring stories, and a list of steps for moving from patient to person as well as treatment info and clinical trials information.

Contact: Joni (916-652-8189) or email @ acpagroups@theacpa.org

Check out "This is Pain" campaign @thisispain or www.thisispain.com, sponsored by ACPA. You will see my story featured.

Free monthly support groups in Austin/Pflugerville, Texas. For meeting info, email my account below. If there is no local support group in your area, consider starting your own. Future online groups coming in 2020.

---

info@chronicpainhacker.com

South Austin- meets 2nd Wednesday of every month at 11 a.m. at Holy Cross Lutheran at 4622 S. Lamar, Austin TX 78745

North Austin- meets last Thursday of every month at 6:30 p.m. at Teapioca Lounge 1713 FM 685, Pflugerville, TX 78660

APPENDIX I
SOCIAL MEDIA

Facebook - "ChronicPainHacker"

YouTube - "ChronicPainHacker"

Instragram - "ChronicPainHacker"

Internet - www.chronicpainhacker.com

GBS/CIDP Foundation International - www.gbs-cidp.org

⋙⋘

Meditation music - Chanting by Dr. Nipun Aggarwal as shown in this link: https://www.youtube.com/watch?v=yoYrLM5rGX8&t=51s

⋙⋘

Energy music - The next song I recommend is binaural beats called "Happiness Frequency" as shown in the link below for meditation and healing: https://www.youtube.com/watch?v=LFGsZ6ythQQ

⋙⋘

Spiritual podcast - "The Next Right Thing" by Emily P Freeman's. This is Christian based but does provide good information for improved decision making and reduced anxiety: www.emilypfreeman.com/podcast/

⋙⋘

Spiritual podcast - "Things Above" by Bryan James Smith called for "mind discipleship": https://apprenticeinstitute.org

⋙⋘

Psychiatrist Directory - Find a licensed psychiatrist in the U.S.:
https://www.psychologytoday.com/us/psychiatrists

۶&

Seton Mind Institute - Located in Austin Texas 512-324-3380
(Psychiatrist Dr. Latham H. Fink):
https://www.seton.net/brain-and-spine-care/

۶&

APEX Manual Therapy - Dr. Alicia Shugart Davis-orthopedic physical
therapy. She has many YouTube videos on posture and PT exercises
to relieve pain. She is amazing! https://www.apexmanualtherapy.com/

۶&

Ice packs - www.accurategelpacks.com or 1-800-660-4972
(these stay cold the longest, come in several sizes, and are affordable)

۶&

Inspirational book - "High Performance Habits" by Brendon Buchard
(book about habits and mantras)

۶&

Gratitude journal - Printable sheet by Sage Grayson at:
www.sagegrayson.com

۶&

Inspirational movie series - "The Kindness Diaries" on Netflix will give
a person perspective on how blessed we truly are. A great series to
watch with your entire family.

۶&

Self improvement - "The Work" by Bryon Katie (free printable work-
sheets for examining your thoughts that teaches a method of self inquiry):
http://thework.com/instruction-the-work-byron-katie/

۶&

Brainspotting - www.goodtherapy.org

જ્વ

Measured count breathing:
https://www.youtube.com/watch?v=WjXnSSRNsWI

જ્વ

Footwear - Brooks shoes can also be purchased at Dick's Sporting goods or online at: https://www.brooksrunning.com

જ્વ

Skechers - Shoes can be purchased at Ross, Amazon or local Skecher store or at: https://www.skechers.com

જ્વ

Acupuncture pen - Piezo Pulse Stimulator (this brand isn't sold on Amazon but there are some more affordable options there): https://www.momentum98.com/piezo.htm

જ્વ

Inspirational speech - Actor Jim Carrey's 2014 commencement speech: https://www.youtube.com/watch?v=V80-gPkpH6M

જ્વ

Infrared heat lamp:
https://www.amazon.com/Beurer-Infrared-Increases-Circulation-IL50/dp/B00IVPMZKE/ref=sr_1_4?crid=TGRY7WDP-314C&keywords=infrared+light+therapy&qid=1552065901&s=gate-way&sprefix=infrared%2Caps%2C188&sr=8-4

જ્વ

PNES information: www.nonepilepticseizures.com

જ્વ

Facebook support group - Psychogenic non epileptic seizures/ conversion disorder support/chat group: www.facebook.com

෧

Clinical Trials Information - https://clinicaltrials.gov/ https://www.findmecure.com

෧

American Physical Therapy Association - 10 pool exercises https://www.moveforwardpt.com/resources/detail/ top-10-exercises-to-do-in-pool

෧

The Body Keeps The Score - Dr. Bessel Van Der Kolk discusses how trauma reshapes the brain and body and offers hope for reclaiming lives.

APPENDIX II

SUPPORT GROUP MEETING NOTES

DATE	ATTENDEES	CONTACT INFO	COMMENTS

DATE	ATTENDEES	CONTACT INFO	COMMENTS

DATE	ATTENDEES	CONTACT INFO	COMMENTS

NOTES

1. Electronic Health Reporter, *accessed March 21, 2020,*
    https://electronichealthreporter.com/the-global-healthcare-crisis/

2. *Colino, Stacey.*"How to Manage Chronic Pain." *Brain and Life Magazine, August/*
    September 2018, Accessed March 21, 2020. https://webdev.brainandlife.org/
    the-magazine/august-september-2018/

3. *Bible Gateway,* accessed March 21, 2020, https://www.biblegateway.com/
    passage/?search=Romans+8%3A28&version=KJV

4. **Realistic Recovery, accessed March 21, 2020,**
    https://www.realisticrecovery.wordpress.com/2009/05/11/
    how-and-why-we-use-19-common-defense-mechanisms/

5. *Good Therapy,* accessed March 21, 2020, https://www.goodtherapy.org/
    learn-about-therapy/types/brainspotting-therapy

6. *HuffPost,* accessed March 21, 2020, https://www.huffpost.com/entry/
    affirmations_b_3527028

7. Linehan, Marsha, *DBT Skills Training Manual 2nd edition*, (New York City, NY;
    Guilford Press, 2015), 14.

8. *Outofstress*, accessed March 21, 2020, https://www.outofstress.com/
    meditation-prefrontal-cortex/

9. *Cleveland Clinic*, accessed March 21, 2020, https://my.clevelandclinic.org/
    health/diagnostics/17479-skin-biopsy-for-small-fiber-sensory-neuropathy

10. *Brain and Life Magazine*, accessed March 21, 2020, https://www.brainandlife.
    org/articles/chronic-pain-doesnt-go-away-but-treating-it-wisely-and/

11. *YouTube "Why Hitting Snooze Ruins Your Brain"*, accessed March 21, 2020,
    https://www.youtube.com/watch?v=iwollxDAmOY

12. *Vice*, accessed March 21, 2020, https://www.vice.com/en_us/article/xwjmpj/
    cbd-drug-test

13. *Wikipedia*, accessed March 21, 2020, https://en.wikipedia.org/wiki/Bloodletting

14. *Telegraph, U.K.*, accessed March 21, 2020, https://
    www.telegraph.co.uk/science/2018/04/27/
    jack-nicklaus-among-first-try-30-stem-cell-therapy-now-plays/

15. *Medtronic*, accessed March 21, 2020, https://www.medtronic.com/us-en/
    healthcare-professionals/therapies-procedures/neurological/spinal-cord-
    stimulation/education-training/about-the-therapy.html

16. *American Migraine Foundation*, accessed March 21, 2020,
    https://americanmigrainefoundation.org/resource-library/
    what-to-know-about-the-new-anti-cgrp-migraine-treatment-options/

17. NIH (National Institute of Neurological Disorders, accessed March 21, 2020, https://www.ninds.nih.gov/disorders/patient-caregiver-education/fact-sheets/guillain-barr%C3%A9-syndrome-fact-sheet#3139_1

18. *KabaFusion*, accessed March 21, 2020, https://kabafusion.com/home-infusion-therapyivig/

19. *Healthline*, accessed March 21, 2020, https://www.healthline.com/health/plasmapheresis

20. *Mayoclinic*, accessed March 2, 2020, https://www.mayoclinic.org/diseases-conditions/guillain-barre-syndrome/diagnosis-treatment/drc-20363006

21. *Psychogenic Non Epileptic Seizures*, accessed March 21, 2020, https://nonepilepticseizures.com/epilepsy-psychogenic-NES-faqs-traumatic-experiences.php

22. *YouTube "Mel Robbins: 5 Second Rule*, accessed March 21, 2020, https://www.youtube.com/watch?v=nl2VQ-ZsNr0

23. *YouTube "Mel Robbins: "Why Motivation is Garbage"*, accessed March 21, 2020, https://www.youtube.com/watch?v=X54GQFS_ouM

ACKNOWLEDGEMENTS

I would like to thank Pat who believed in my noble effort.

I would like to thank Dr. Fink for helping me regain my confidence.

I would like to thank my amazing primary physician Dr. Chau Nguyen, M.D. who goes above and beyond and his colleague, Dr. Alicia Shugart Davis, DPT. Together they provide integrated medicine that treats the whole person. I love them so much that my entire family sees them.

I would like to thank Dr. James Dean, M.D,. Neurology. Your early detection and treatment gave me a second chance.

I would like to thank Dr. Elizabeth Peckham, D.O., Neurology for your compassionate care and open discussion of integrated medicine.

I would like to thank Amber C., LMT, for making house calls and providing massage with cupping and graston techniques and most of all for her friendship.

I would like to thank Michael Parrish, LMT, for making a CBD based pain relief cream that is the best on the market.

I would like to thank Pree Poonati, personal trainer and yoga master. I have gratitude for the practice of meditation and mindfulness at Nirvana Gym.

I would like to thank Chaz Wesley for helping me find my "why" again.

I would like to thank Carol for helping me understand "radical acceptance".

I would like to thank Renee Fisher, my publisher, for helping this dream come true.

I would like to thank God for his deliverance out of the wilderness.

I would like to thank my husband and son who have my back.

Shannon Green

ABOUT THE AUTHOR

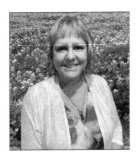 Shannon Green Shannon Green is a chronic pain expert and support group facilitator for the American Chronic Pain Association. Shannon is originally from Bartlesville, Oklahoma but resides in Austin, Texas with her husband, son, and fur babies. Her passion is supporting the chronic pain community and improving healthcare standards and legislation. Shannon loves creating mixed media art in her studio and making handmade greeting cards. She is a graduate of Oklahoma State University with an MBA from Oklahoma City University.

Follow her at @chronicpainhacker on Instagram, Facebook, and YouTube